Mayview O.T.

MAYVIEW STATE HOSPITAL
BRIDGEVILLE, PA. 15017

Therapeutic Activities for the Handicapped Elderly

Charlotte M. Hamill, M.A., M.S.S.W.
Associate Director for Planning
and Program Development
Burke Rehabilitation Center
White Plains, New York

Robert C. Oliver, M.A.
Associate Professor of Psychology
Pace University
New York, New York

With special contributions from
Nancy Benes, O.T.R.
and
Ann Krieger

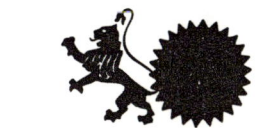

AN ASPEN PUBLICATION®
Aspen Systems Corporation
Rockville, Maryland
London
1980

Library of Congress Cataloging in Publication Data

Hamill, Charlotte M.
Therapeutic activities for the handicapped elderly.

Bibliographies: p. 255, p. 283
Includes index.

1. Aged—Rehabilitation. 2. Handicapped—Rehabilitation. 3. Occupational therapy. I. Oliver, Robert C., joint author. II. Title. [DNLM: 1. Occupational therapy—In old age. 2. Handicapped. WB555 H217t]
RC952.5.H34   615.8'515   80-19661
ISBN: 0-89443-326-1

Copyright © 1980 by Aspen Systems Corporation

All rights reserved. This book, or parts thereof, may not be reproduced in any form or by any means, electronic or mechanical, including photocopy, recording, or any information storage and retrieval system now known or to be invented, without written permission from the publisher, except in the case of brief quotations embodied in critical articles or reviews. For information, address Aspen Systems Corporation, 1600 Research Boulevard, Rockville, Maryland, 20850.

Library of Congress Catalog Card Number: 80-19661
ISBN: 0-89443-326-1

Printed in the United States of America

1 2 3 4 5

To Priscilla Adams
whose creativity, commitment, and concern for individuals
inspired us to produce this book.

Table of Contents

Foreword ix

Acknowledgments xi

    PART I 1

Chapter 1—The Therapeutic Approach 3

    Uses of Activities 3
    Analysis of Activities 4
    Types of Activities 5
    Evaluation of Participants 5

Chapter 2—Group Activities 25

    Formation of Groups 26
    Operation of Groups 26
    Group Projects 27

Chapter 3—Motivating Participants 29

    Motivation Methods 30
    Problems in Motivating 30

Chapter 4—Operating the Program 33

    Keys to Effectiveness 33
    Typical Activities 34
    Program Structure 35
    Education for Staff 36

Chapter 5—The Use of Volunteers 39

    Recruitment and Motivation 40
    Selection and Orientation 41
    Training 42
    Assignment 42
    Potential Problems 43

Chapter 6—The Facility 47

    Important Factors 47
    Floors 48
    Doors 49
    Windows 49
    Tables 49
    Chairs 49
    Ventilation 50
    Storage Units 50
    Bathrooms 50
    Basins 51
    Useful Items 51

Chapter 7—Equipment and Supplies 53

    Use of Discarded Materials 53
    Expensive Items 54
    Borrowing 54
    Safety 55
    Organization of Equipment and Supplies 55
    Cautions 57
    Summary 57

Chapter 8—A News Publication 59

    Essentials 59
    Benefits 60
    Successful Methods 60

Chapter 9—Food Preparation by Participants 63

    Goals 64
    Choices 65
    Kitchen Features 66

Table of Contents

Chapter 10—Carry-over to the Home 67
    Practical Use of Abilities 67
    Family Assistance 68
    Transportation 68
    The Community 69

PART II 71

Chapter 11—Therapeutic Craft Activities 73

Chapter 12—Projects for the Visually Impaired or Blind 75
    Working with the Multi-handicapped 75
    The Isolated Person 77
    Braille, Large Type, and Recordings 78

Chapter 13—Craft Projects 79
    Paper and Glue 79
    Printing and Stationery 97
    Braid Weaving and Turkish Knotting 105
    String Art 113
    Yarn Winding 121
    Stitchery 127
    Leather Lacing 155
    Batik and Tie Dyeing 163
    Decorative Containers 169
    Art 179
    Mosaics 183
    Modeling with Clay, Dough, and Cornstarch 189
    Flowers 207
    Nature Materials 215
    Horticulture 229
    Woodworking 233

Bibliography—General 255

Appendix A—Aids for Daily Living 257

Appendix B—Activity Equipment 261

Appendix C—Craft Supply Companies 267

Appendix D—Food-Preparation Equipment for the Disabled 271

Appendix E—Aids for the Visually Impaired 275

Appendix F—Magazines 279

Appendix G—Medical Glossary 281

Bibliography—Crafts 283

Index 287

Foreword

The increase in longevity has brought with it a rise in the nation's chronically ill and physically disabled. Current estimates put their number at 20 million, of whom some 40 percent are 65 or older.

Many of the elderly population are functionally impaired and require care and support to continue living in their communities independently. In 1973, a new option came into being which demonstrated that in many instances older people with incapacitating illness could be treated and cared for during the day, thus avoiding or at least postponing institutionalization or custodial care and substantially reducing the isolation that accompanies remaining at home alone. This new option was the Day Hospital, a division of the Burke Rehabilitation Center in White Plains, New York. The Burke program began as a research demonstration project funded by the U.S. Department of Health, Education, and Welfare. Its services were medically oriented, with strong psychosocial components. It was the experience with one of these components, the therapeutic activities program, that served as the impetus for this handbook.

These therapeutic activities provide social interaction, a wide range of handicrafts and games, and mental and aesthetic stimulation. The Day Hospital staff found the activities to be particularly effective in reinforcing the residual strengths and meeting the psychosocial needs of handicapped persons. Also, it became apparent that while therapeutic activities were an integral part of the Day Hospital treatment they could be carried on independently in a variety of other settings. The activities were especially helpful to chronically ill, physically disabled older persons in counteracting isolation, restoring self-confidence and self-esteem, and improving personal relationships.

A therapeutic activities program for handicapped adults need not have the sophisticated facilities or highly trained professional staff of a day hospital such as Burke's. It can be organized by lay persons, with the assistance of a professional staff or consultants. It can be related to a senior citizens center, a service club, a nutrition program, a church's community service program, a hospital, a social agency outreach program, a stroke club, etc.

The activities, for the most part, are familiar ones but are specifically adapted, often in fairly simple ways, for the handicapped. Considerable use is made of group projects—even for groups whose members have differing handicaps and abilities—and the results are often of such quality as to engender pride. The activity groups are designed to provide the right kind of exercise, either mental or physical, for each participant. The underlying goal is not to weave a basket, for example, but to improve one's coordination. Two people, each weaving a basket, may be presented with this task in two different ways, for the special kind of therapy each person needs. In the purely recreational activities, as in those that are more imaginative and innovative, the goal is therapy, and the individually prescribed activities are the key to success.

Therapy has many facets. This handbook focuses on activities that are basically psychosocial and that increase the abilities of the participants or improve their feelings of self-worth and independence. Part I discusses philosophy, principles, and procedures. Part II provides specific instructions for a wide range of activities, with special emphasis on their therapeutic effects for various disabilities.

Acknowledgments

This book represents the efforts and contributions of many individuals and organizations. It was inspired by the success of a unique therapeutic activities program in an adult day hospital. The creativity and artistic talents of the paid and volunteer staff members resulted in several educational and training programs and requests for written materials.

The therapeutic activities program was developed under the leadership of Priscilla Adams, who also assisted in the initial stages of the manuscript development. Professional supervision and guidance for the program was provided by Nancy Benes, O.T.R., who also was a major contributor to the book. The endless work involved in developing ideas for activities and in describing projects with words and sketches was carefully and skillfully coordinated by Ann Krieger.

It would be impossible to enumerate the contributions of all who helped, but some brief comments are in order. Ideas, projects, clinical adaptations, and sketches were contributed by Harriet Dandridge, Charles Darville, Tommie Davis, Joan Gross, Geri Helfer, Avis Hofstad, Elsa McAvoy, Margo Meyer, Gene Reed, and Maureen Ryan—all paid staff members and volunteers in our day hospital program. The staff is especially appreciative of the art work contributed by Barbara Goodman, a professional artist who so generously donated her time and talents. Technical editorial assistance for certain chapters was provided by Barbara Carter and Gloria Dapper. Consultation was provided also by Helen Proctor and Elizabeth Lincoln. Final editing and manuscript preparation were coordinated by Milica Dingwall with the assistance of Edna Fernandez, Carole Haber, and Elizabeth Mercer.

The patients who participated in the day hospital were the real inspiration for the staff members who developed the many projects. The continuing interest and requests of visiting professionals encouraged the sharing of results of the team's efforts. It is hoped that staff and participants in other institutions will benefit from these materials and will adapt them to meet their particular needs.

Part I

Chapter 1

The Therapeutic Approach

The subject of this handbook is the therapeutic programming of craft activities. The purpose of therapeutic, in contrast to diversional, activities is to stimulate changes in the participants' abilities from dysfunctional to functional. Activities to accomplish this must be selected to meet each individual's physical and psychosocial needs. This process is different from that of a recreation program, where the primary emphasis is on providing pleasure for the participants. Recreational activities may produce innately therapeutic rewards and increased capabilities. If they are directed toward those goals, they would probably be described as "therapeutic recreation."

USES OF ACTIVITIES

The handicraft activities presented in this volume could be well utilized in a therapeutic recreation program. They have been used successfully for disabled individuals and groups of varying ages (but primarily adults), and can also be enjoyed by non-handicapped persons. Disabilities of the participants in these activities cover a broad range, with a predominance of long-term chronic illnesses and handicapping conditions.

The program was designed to meet three primary goals:

1. improvement of function to the degree possible
2. prevention of deterioration
3. utilization of the participant's residual abilities.

The range of an activity program should be determined by the physical and mental abilities of the participants and the aim must always be to increase their independence. Activities must also have relevance for the individual in his day-to-day social environment. Individual goals must be clearly stated, and performance must be supervised to ensure that the selected activities meet each participant's needs.

ANALYSIS OF ACTIVITIES

For achieving therapeutic goals, each activity must be analyzed for its psychological and physical components by breaking it down and analyzing the abilities required in each step. The activities must be capable of gradation, to provide for different physical and mental capability, and they must have continuity (e.g., one active motion of hand opening is useless if the remainder of the activity calls for static positioning of the hand). The activities must allow adaptation, either in simplifying a task or increasing its complexity. They must also have a conclusion and a means of judging performance and monitoring effectiveness.

Some participants may require sessions (to include specific exercises) with a trained therapist, either individually or in a group. However, the therapeutic effects of the activities described here can serve as a reinforcement to abilities being redeveloped. It may not be realistic to attempt to improve the physical or mental abilities of some persons, in light of their irreversible deficits. Utilizing residual skills should then become the program's primary objective.

One or more of the following goals may be met through a therapeutic activity program:

- Assist the person to compensate for physical loss (e.g., one-handed skill training).
- Use avocational outlets, appropriate to the individual's limitations, to meet the need to be useful and productive.
- Assist in the adaptation of environment to allow more functional independence.
- Increase safety awareness for those with a sensory, perceptual, or cognitive loss.
- Increase perceptual awareness.
- Help the participant to cope with loss by providing opportunities for achievement.
- Utilize residual intellectual capabilities through activities that stimulate orientation, concentration, decision making, and problem solving.
- Help the individual improve social facility to improve personal relationships.

- Increase the participant's potential for a satisfying role in the community (home, family, friends, civic involvement).

TYPES OF ACTIVITIES

Exhibits 1-1 through 1-4 list a variety of disabilities in four categories—social-psychological, physical, sensory, and perceptual—to give some direction in setting goals and some general ideas for appropriate activities. The social-psychological problems are given first, as such difficulties affect motivation, on which everything else depends. The comments in the charts are keys to helping ensure individual success. Disease categories have not been mentioned, because the resulting disabilities vary widely. It should not be presumed that the activities listed are the only possible choices; the comments and goals, however, are specific to the deficit listed.

Each activity makes its own unique therapeutic contributions, as will be discussed in detail later in this book. Some activities provide latitude to move in many directions, and not all of the participants will achieve the same end results.

EVALUATION OF PARTICIPANTS

How does one evaluate the effectiveness of the activity, or the program as a whole, for an individual? Documentation is one of the essentials for assessing progress and determining whether activities are appropriate and goals are being achieved. The size and type of the facility, the nature of the participants, the program budget, and the number of staff supervisors will determine what kind of recording is necessary and feasible.

Although objective testing may be done by the professional staff, important information may be added by paraprofessionals, who may be in closer contact with the participants. This is especially true for psychosocial factors. The sample profile, Exhibit 1-5, is to be used by the paraprofessional staff to augment more specific testing.

Before setting up a means of recording, it is essential to determine the kind of information desired, the skills of the staff members making the assessment, and the use to which the information will be put. A form that is kept in a specific place with limited access to other staff members has little value other than to the few who are doing the recording. A check form, such as the sample shown in Exhibit 1-5, can be useful, not only in helping the staff analyze participant performance, but in assisting them in analyzing components of the activities. It can serve as a guide to more formal verbal reporting, such as team conferences.

Exhibit 1-1 Social-Psychological Difficulties

DIFFICULTY	GOALS	HELPFUL KINDS OF ACTIVITIES	COMMENTS
1. Reactive depression, evidenced by withdrawal or non-participation in response to a handicap or loss (not usually requiring psychiatric treatment)	Increased motivation to participate in life, and lifting of the depression	Activities that encourage the expression of feelings (discussion groups, newsletters, art, music, dramatic skits).	Caution: don't force a reluctant person to express opinions or participate openly in a group. Let it come naturally. Just watching from the sidelines may be enough for a time.
		Activities that provide opportunities to see how others are coping with disabilities, and to share feelings and problems.	
	Renewed interest in life	Activities that draw on a person's interests or experiences (travels, hobbies, regional or ethnic contributions to history, occupation—e.g., a baker may ice cupcakes for a party; a violinist may bring records for a session on music appreciation).	
	Less preoccupation with self		

		Activities that introduce the person to new experiences that may uncover hidden talent (painting, gardening, sewing, woodworking, etc.) or offer mental stimulation along with companionship.	
2. Low self-esteem	Increased sense of self-worth	Activities in which the person can experience success, either in learning or relearning something or in contributing to the group.	Choose activities at a level that will ensure success without demeaning the participant.
	Increased sense of self-confidence	Activities that not only ensure success but show a measure of progress, however minute.	May require grading activities, moving from the easier steps to the more complicated, so that the person can feel involved in a significant, however small, degree in a worthwhile project.
	Increased appreciation of residual capabilities	Activities that reduce the feeling of dependency by furthering self-care abilities (eating, dressing, etc.) and homemaking (ordering groceries, arranging for cleaning, etc.).	See Appendixes A and D for aids in ADL and food preparation.

Exhibit 1-1 continued

DIFFICULTY	GOALS	HELPFUL KINDS OF ACTIVITIES	COMMENTS
		Activities that introduce the participant to the wide variety of things possible—especially those that can be continued at home or independently—and that invite continued pursuit (horticulture and gardening, sewing and needlework, cooking and bread-making, painting, music, card games and table games, bird watching, carpentry).	Requires scheduling the hours of each person's day on a chart to provide variety, maintain interest, preclude fatigue, and balance possible frustrations with successes. Caution: While a schedule is necessary, it should not be rigid; revisions should be allowed and a choice of activities permitted.
	Increased recognition that the person is doing something important that is appreciated by someone else	Arrange shows of participants' art work, crafts, garden displays, and Christmas decorations in libraries, hospitals, theaters, boutiques, the state capitol, legislative offices. Arrange ways to ensure recognition of contributions to a group project (toasts, mention in a newsletter, citations, display).	

		Increased participation in the mainstream of life	Activities a person might hesitate to do alone (e.g., taking a small group out to a restaurant or the theater, or to the "Y" for swimming during a reserved hour). Activities of recognized social value (helping to plan an in-house party, a telephone campaign to help find summer jobs for the unemployed, preparing simple learning materials for retarded children, etc.).	
3. Damaged self-image (not to be confused with distorted body image; see Exhibit 1-4, No. 2)		Increased adaptation to the situation and acceptance of self as-is	Activities that provide a person with the opportunity to take the lead, to be on the giving end, and to receive positive recognition by other members of the group.	Caution: Do not use expressions such as "bad arm," "bad side," etc. Make access to these opportunities as easy as possible, and avoid unnecessary waiting and frustration.
4. Short concentration span; poor memory		Prevention of further loss, increased use of memory in daily activities, and increased ability to make simple decisions	Activities that range from simple memory games (matching cards or shapes) to somewhat more involved activities that require management of time sequences and a shift from task to task to achieve a goal	Requires • a narrow range of choices • carefully structured (step-by-step) activities involving repetitive procedures

Exhibit 1-1 continued

DIFFICULTY	GOALS	HELPFUL KINDS OF ACTIVITIES	COMMENTS
		(e.g., window gardening, from choice of plants and pots, through planting and watering, to watching growth).	• carefully graded activities that move easily from one level of difficulty to the next • a carefully structured environment—low-key, free of distractions (people, noise, unnecessary supplies) Folding screens may be used to set off a quiet place.
5. Confusion; disorientation	Increased orientation to reality; more awareness of time, place, and people	Activities that involve constant reference to familiar or necessary things and people, such as games to name parts of the body with 3, 4, or 5 letters; to identify objects drawn from a bag or pictures of items of daily use; to make or finish sentences; to work simple puzzles.	Requires giving one direction at a time, and perhaps demonstration of the written or verbal instructions. May require individual attention, with daily reminders of day, names, time, and activities. Large calendars and clocks are important. Note: This illustrates the importance of staff members wearing name tags.
6. Inability to communicate basic needs	Increased verbal or nonverbal communication	Activities (similar to those in No. 5) for the partially verbal that stimulate or support verbalization of basic needs.	Referral to a speech therapist may be indicated, with activities designed to reinforce progress made.

The Therapeutic Approach 11

		Activities for the nonverbal that develop gestures and body language, and group activities in which they can participate (singing, gardening, etc.).	This may require demonstrations to those at home or close to the patient. Note: "Nonverbal" does not mean that a patient does not understand.
7. Disruptive behavior (anger, throwing cards in the air, etc.)	Stop the disruptive behavior and help the person show emotion in a socially acceptable manner	After responding directly to the behavior ("I can see you are disturbed, unhappy, uncomfortable . . ."): • Shift to more quiet activities (listening to music, having a snack joining a different group—whatever is within the person's abilities and non-threatening). • Or shift to an activity in which the participant can work off emotions (carpentry, rolling clay, hammering metal, etc.)	Caution: All behavior has meaning, and may well be appropriate to the stress. While disruptive behavior must be stopped, the cause is important, and may require learning about the person's physical and emotional life at home to interpret behavior with understanding, in order to deal with it appropriately.
8. Inappropriate behavior, such as weeping or laughing, when no cause is evident	Help the person achieve control over behavior	May require moving the person to quieter activities without attracting the attention of the group.	Note: Crying may indicate pain or sadness, or it may be the result of brain damage affecting emotional control.

Exhibit 1-1 continued

DIFFICULTY	GOALS	HELPFUL KINDS OF ACTIVITIES	COMMENTS
9. Hyperactivity, wandering, unable to keep still	Direct energy into a safe activity	Short-term, well-structured activities, interspersed with gross motor activities (e.g., dancing, Ping-Pong, throwing quoits, catching balls or balloons).	Caution: Close supervision is required if sharp tools, hot equipment, or abrasive materials are used.

The Therapeutic Approach

Exhibit 1-2 Physical Disabilities

DISABILITY	GOALS	HELPFUL KINDS OF ACTIVITIES	COMMENTS
1. Loss of leg or legs	Increased or maintained strength throughout, especially in the upper extremities (if the central problem is distorted body image, see Exhibit 1-4, No. 2)	Many activities are appropriate (including garden hoeing, lawn bowling, horseshoe pitching, and shuffleboard for those in a wheelchair). If the person is ambulatory, encourage walking.	Amputees may have complicating problems, such as diabetes or loss of sensation (see Exhibit 1-3, No. 4).
2. Loss of function or motion in one hand or arm	Prevention of joint immobility or further damage of the affected part	Any activity that allows the affected arm or hand to be supported on a table or rested comfortably on a lap board or pillow to maintain good joint mobility	Good positioning is important. Caution: Exercise of extremely lax muscles, or those that exhibit spasticity, should be supervised only by a trained therapist.
	Increased ability of the other hand, or shift in dominance	Almost all activities can be adapted for the one-handed person, working either alone or with another person.	Require stabilizing or holding devices, such as table clamps, clipboards, vises, tape, weights, one-handed needle-threaders (see Appendix B), anchored spindles for yarn, etc.
		Activities that can be done easily with one hand, such as card or board games.	The person may tend to ignore the affected side (evidenced by work completed on one side

Exhibit 1-2 continued

DISABILITY	GOALS	HELPFUL KINDS OF ACTIVITIES	COMMENTS
		Crafts that do not require stablizing devices, such as shell craft, small flat pinecone projects, clay projects.	only) and may need to be repositioned. Those close to the person at home may need to be informed of the problem and of positioning techniques.
		Crafts that can be clamped for one-handed work (e.g., embroidery, needlepoint, leather-lacing).	
3. Limited use of muscle or joint	Maintained or increased strength and range of motion in the affected area	Repetitive activities should be used for both gross and fine muscles, graded step by step in strength, coordination, and range of motion, from those requiring assistance to light but unassisted tasks (such as picking up light objects) to those requiring some force against resistance (sanding, filing, etc.).	Caution: Despite the attention paid to disabilities, the main focus must never be the arm or leg, but the whole person.
	Improvement in hip, knee, or ankle	Activities involving treadles and foot levers (potter's wheel, floor loom, piano, etc.).	

Improvement in shoulder	Activities such as braiding, or weaving, lacing (to increase the range of motion, discourage lap work; use slant boards, easels, or longer lacings to encourage reaching), sanding, sawing, ceramics, shuffleboard, horseshoes.	
Improvement in forearms	Same as for the shoulder, plus twisting (wire jewelry, decorative screws, etc.)	
Improvement in wrist	Many of the previous activities, plus hammering (e.g., metal ashtrays), stencilling, rolling clay, etc.	Damp clay may affect joints. Substitute bread dough if necessary.
Improvement in hands and fingers	Activities that require frequent grasping and releasing (punching, cutting, weaving, cord knotting, clay modeling, making pinch pots, piano playing, typing, etc.)	Arthritics with hand involvement should be discouraged from using fine hand tools, such as knitting needles or crochet hooks, for a protracted length of time. Activities requiring frequent opening and closing of the hand (e.g., cutting) are better. Tools may require built-up handles made of bicycle handle grips, foam rubber, screw-on wooden handles, or dowels.

Exhibit 1-2 continued

DISABILITY	GOALS	HELPFUL KINDS OF ACTIVITIES	COMMENTS
			Caution: It may not be possible to improve dexterity with some disabilities. If not, do not frustrate the person with fine motor activities such as sewing or beading.
4. Limited endurance	Avoidance of fatigue, and increased ability to participate in activities for longer periods	Most activities of short duration and scheduled for the person's best time (the morning may be best for those with muscle weakness or coordination problems; afternoon is frequently better for many arthritics).	Gradually increase the length of time of activities and the grade, from light to heavier. The program should be adapted for patients with limited endurance. Those with cardiac limitations should be supervised closely for shortness of breath and changes in color or temperature
5. Lack of muscle coordination	Compensation for loss Maintained or increased coordination	Gross, non-exacting activities (magnetic board games, sanding, rolling clay). Light activities not requiring fine coordination (decoupage, stencilling, etc.)	As with lack of endurance, short activities are best. May require a limited work space (marked off with tongue depressors, wood strips, or tape, or placed in a shallow box) and stabilizers (clamps, weights, florist's clay, or Scotch tape)

			Uncoordinated participants may be able to function better in verbal-discussion group games.
6. Lack of head-trunk control	Utilization of residual control	Verbalization groups, games, play acting, and music groups.	If the trunk is uncoordinated, it may require stabilizing with a restrainer or pillows, or the person may have better control of the hands when the arms are kept close to the body.
7. Inability to initiate motion	Bring the person into activities and help move from one activity to another	Automatic, repetitive activities are often best (ball-playing, Ping-Pong, sanding, etc.)	Don't force a person to move, but provide the stimulus to move when the person indicates interest.
		Balance physical activities with discussion and conversation groups as well as word games.	Give short, direct verbal cues when initiating activity.
			The inability to begin movement is not necessarily related to the loss of muscle power, but may be associated with a dysfunction that affects the stimulus to move. When the sensory system is bombarded with stimulating input (e.g., a ball is thrown at one), a protective response is often elicited (e.g., one moves to stop the ball or push it away).

Exhibit 1-3 Sensory Disabilities

DISABILITY	GOALS	HELPFUL KINDS OF ACTIVITIES	COMMENTS
1. Diminished vision or blindness	Compensation for loss	Depending on the extent of impairment: • activities using strong color contrasts (braiding with different colors, weaving with color-cued warp, etc.) • tactile activities (ceramics, one-color glazing, pine cone projects, Turkish knotting, knitting with short needles, etc.) • aromatic activities (windowsill herb garden, potpourri bags, etc.) • language activities (conversation, being read to, sing-alongs, dramatic skits, talking books, large-type books)	May require orienting participants to the room and work materials by touch—by letting them feel a completed example of the project first, by limiting work space, and by using tactile guidelines for work (cloth markers, measuring tape stapled to indicate inches and feet, etc.). See Chapter 12.
Loss of visual field	Increased awareness of what part of the visual field is missing, and helping the person compensate	The choice of activities will be dependent upon the extent of impairment.	Position objects at first where the person can see easily, but gradually move them to the affected area to encourage the use of head movement in compensation.

2. Loss of hearing, deafness	Increased participant awareness of loss and helping participant compensate	Most activities are possible. Rhythm bands are good.	May require non-verbal instructions or demonstrations, or seating a person with the best ear toward the group, or facing a person who is a lip reader. Caution: Those wearing hearing aids may be very sensitive to sharp, loud noises (hammering, etc.). They may inadvertently dislodge or disconnect their hearing aids. Check to see if the hearing aid is working.
3. Loss of speech	Increased verbalization (if possible) and increased comprehension of language Increased participation in social activities Communication by means other than language	Activities that encourage both written and oral communication (morning greetings, sing-alongs, simple fill-in-the-word games, copying, writing, reading with a ruler, matching tasks such as word-to-picture, word-to-word, etc.). Activities that foster communication through writing, typing, use of an alphabet board, gestures, etc.	May require referral to a speech therapist and activities designed to support the therapy. It is useful to display a picture board of activities of daily living for basic needs.
4. Loss of sensation—touch, taste, or sensitivity to hot or cold	Improvement of sensation or compensation for loss	Activities that offer a variety of tactile sensations (see No. 1 in this exhibit) and opportunity for increased discrimination.	Caution: May require increasing the person's awareness of loss to safeguard against accidents, especially from caustic or irritating chemicals (turpentine, oil-base paints, etc.), sharp tools, and bumping of extremities.

Exhibit 1-4 Perceptual Disabilities

DISABILITY	GOALS	HELPFUL KINDS OF ACTIVITIES	COMMENTS
1. Loss of ability to interpret sensory experiences —in seeing	Compensation for loss, increased perceptual awareness, and, where necessary, increased ability to organize and plan ahead (see Exhibit 1-1, Nos. 4 and 5)	Activities that involve: • eye-hand coordination (follow simple patterns in mosaic tile setting, leather lacing, embroidery, etc.) • depth perception (three-dimensional puzzles, simple hand weaving, basketry, etc.) • left-right and vertical-horizontal discrimination (weaving, tracing, needlepoint, leather lacing, etc.) • spatial relationships of sizes, colors, textures (collages, nature art, geometric puzzles, etc.) • size constancy (sorting—tiles, fabrics, nuts and bolts—and stacking or pyramiding)	A perceptual difficulty is not a loss of ability in the organ of reception, such as the eye, but rather a defect in the interpretation of sensory experiences. This usually requires a series of relearning experiences to help the person recognize stimuli for what they are (e.g., the use of raised lines to reinforce horizontal and vertical).
—in hearing		Repetitious activities that involve responding with understanding to what is heard (simple question-and-answer phrases, games, craft instructions, etc.).	

—in touching		Activities, with manual guidance, offering repeated practice with familiar objects (spoons, scissors, or coins) or using similar motions (cup and glass, pencil and crayon, etc.). Use materials with different textures to stimulate discrimination.	Note: Material placed around a crochet hook, for example, and molded to the full contour of the person's hand grasp, or a wooden dowel may enable those whose touch is limited to the fingers to hold on to the tool.
2. Distorted body image	Help the person to be aware of body parts and the relation of a specific part to the function of entire body	Activities involving spatial relationships of the body to other persons or objects. Games such as "Simon Says" and "Lubby Loo," or matching of parts of the body. Two-handed activities such as rolling clay, sanding with a two-handed sander, loom weaving, hammering, or beating. Sensory-stimulating activities to promote awareness of body parts (using rough-textured materials, for instance). Activities to promote awareness of the relationships between body parts (e.g., completing drawings of person, tracing body templates).	Skills acquired in this area will particularly benefit self-care abilities.

Exhibit 1-5 Therapeutic Activities Participant Profile

Participant _____ Code: 3—always
                                                                                     2—sometimes
                                                                                     1—never
                                                                                     x—not observed

CODE	OBSERVATION	COMMENTS
	Physical	
_____	Has good gross coordination.	
_____	Has good dexterity.	
_____	Uses residual abilities well.	
_____	Has good endurance for activities.	
_____	Has good vision.	
_____	Is competent with tools and equipment.	
	Mental	
_____	Is well-oriented.	
_____	Is consistent in performance.	
_____	Has good perception.	
_____	Has good attention span.	
_____	Follows directions without repetition.	
_____	Shows good comprehension of visual directions.	
_____	Demonstrates good safety awareness.	
	Social	
_____	Relates well to staff members.	
_____	Socializes with other participants.	
_____	Helps other participants (as able).	
_____	Participates in activities.	
	Emotional	
_____	Is emotionally stable.	
_____	Is self-confident.	
	Initiative	
_____	Initiates own projects.	
_____	Makes own decisions about projects.	
	General	
_____	Is interested in a variety of activities.	
_____	Completes projects.	
_____	Follows the rules.	
_____	Shows good carry-over to the home.	

Special skills, abilities, and interests noted:

Problems noted:

Date _____ Evaluator _____

A record demonstrating a participant's ability to initiate and carry out activities independently should stimulate the staff to promote that person to activities with more responsibility. The participant whose assessment indicates varying performance from day to day should perhaps be allowed more flexibility in program planning. (For example, if a person's concentration is poor on a particular day, a schedule requiring that person to function in an hour-long craft session would be inappropriate. He or she might better function in an activity that requires less concentration such as a music group or physical game. Flexibility in programming is allowed but structure should be maintained within a group.)

Chapter 2

Group Activities

The group work process is a recognized treatment method for the elderly and functionally impaired, in the form of the reality orientation group, remotivation therapy group, or therapeutic activities group. The focus and the amount of direction may vary, but the same basic principles are applicable. The desirability of participation in a group will depend upon a person's ability to tolerate the group format, to communicate, and to engage in the group tasks. Maintaining groups can be a demanding task for leaders, particularly if they are uneasy with the dependency on them that may develop among the group members. The aim of the group should be to increase the self-confidence of its members and to increase their abilities to sustain personal relationships.

A leader is essential in a group to help set standards, maintain direction, stimulate or channel efforts when necessary, and act as an intermediary when problems occur. Leadership may be assumed by group members. When participants change in the group and leadership roles shift, monitoring by the staff is particularly important.

Support is one of the greatest values a group can offer. Examples of this are: the gifted musician who can no longer play but is urged by group members to share some knowledge by discussing a composer's work along with a music program; the overweight person who is ashamed of letting the group down by cheating on a diet; and the partially paralyzed woman teaching other group members some tricks she has learned in dressing, along with some simple dress alterations.

Sharing problems with others may provide a constructive outlet and make the problems more tolerable. It can stimulate change in the individual's conception of the problem or help in dealing with the difficulty.

FORMATION OF GROUPS

Groups may form spontaneously. For example, participants meeting over coffee and discussing world happenings may decide that they want to meet regularly, giving birth to a weekly current-events group. Or a visiting lecturer from the Audubon Society may stimulate members to make bird houses or study the birds they observe at the facility or their homes, and share with the group what they have learned.

Groups may be short-term, related to a current happening such as a holiday, religious event, or forthcoming election. Members might invite a representative from the League of Women Voters to discuss the voting process. Other members might organize a debate or discussion group or be responsible for getting members to use absentee ballots.

Sometimes a small suggestion can grow into a major project. An example of this in one facility was a group formed to commemorate the Bicentennial, starting from an offhand remark by a participant about doing something special to mark the event. Members were encouraged by the group to bring in clippings, pictures, and memorabilia to post on a bulletin board; others met to design a Bicentennial quilt, featuring early flags. Others studied the history of the flags, while some met to plan a skit featuring Betsy Ross. The interest in history stimulated interest in colonial crafts, such as apple and cornhusk dolls, as well as research into the past for articles to be written in a news publication.

Group involvement is most successful when the impetus has come from the group members, but it is the organizing or supervising staff who must direct these ideas toward goal-related activities. This does not happen without planning and effort.

OPERATION OF GROUPS

The staff must know the group members as individuals in order to work with them effectively in a group. Projects undertaken together must be geared to accommodate each person's disabilities, abilities, and personal interests so all can participate in some way—possibly in the planning and organizing. This calls for activity analysis.

Sessions should be long enough to accomplish something, but not so long as to cause fatigue. More sedentary activities can be saved for later in the day, when group members have less energy. Reasonable time periods should be allowed for group activities (e.g., if a music appreciation group is initiated, it should be able to meet often enough to develop a program). Initial group meetings often set the tone for following sessions, so it is important to plan and promote a successful beginning. Realistic timetables should be set for seasonal group projects. Pressure on groups to accomplish goals by a certain date may detract from the satisfaction of their involvement. However, learning to meet deadlines may be useful in increasing responsibility.

The optimal group size will depend, of course, upon the project, the needs of the individual members, the space available, and the capability of the group leader. Discussion groups are usually more effective when there are eight to ten members. Eight or fewer are best for a craft group containing persons with a variety of disabilities who are working on similar projects. Food preparation groups may function best with four or five if space permits.

Guiding a group calls for tact and diplomacy. Members do not always blend well together. If one member tends to dominate, the others may become dissatisfied. Some group members may not be able to participate or give their views. The capable leader is sensitive to group moods. A domineering leader may be complimented openly, but privately asked for ideas to get the other group members more involved (implying that the aggressive one should step back). Another approach might be for a staff member to shift attention to another member's unique skills by presenting the group with a problem that requires other members' participation. Encouraging group members to be open with one another often provides the necessary groundwork for the members to take more responsibility for controlling themselves.

Some members always tend to sit back and listen. It is the skillful leader who is alert to signs of boredom or of interest (e.g., an uncommunicative person who taps a foot during a music program may be unconsciously giving a clue to an interest in rhythm or sing-along groups.)

Participants may have a need for belonging, for a place in which they can contribute. Some older members may sense rejection and have a feeling of dependence that damages self-esteem. Contributing to group projects that are important to others can help to combat these feelings.

GROUP PROJECTS

Participants may take on a community service project, such as making educational aids for a nursery school or performing a telephone service for schools, such as finding out which companies hire students for vacation periods. Or they may make needed articles for other members (e.g., tote bags for walkers or wheelchairs; card holders, or lapboards). They may write or call local restaurants, stores, or other community facilities to investigate accessibility for the handicapped, and make up a handbook for participants.

All activities based on individual interests lend spontaneity, freshness, and flexibility to the program, but the individual's satisfaction as part of a group depends on what occurs during the process. The most beneficial group activities are those that are based on the interests and abilities of the members and increase their capacity for independence and creativity. The activities described in this chapter have been suggested as possibilities for group work. However, the craft activities described in Part II can be used for either individuals or groups, depending on the abilities, disabilities, and interests of the participants. For some groups, individuals accomplish parts of an activity project and the entire group is responsible for the finished product. In other groups, two persons may share a project while others work individually. Personal interactions are important in all of these settings, and the trained leader utilizes every opportunity to enrich the process.

Chapter 3

Motivating Participants

Once goals have been determined and activities selected, the challenge becomes getting the participants involved. An established program is an impetus in itself to newcomers, since it offers visible evidence of people enjoying what they are doing, an atmosphere of sociability, warmth and concern, and a number of interesting activities in process. Motivation for involvement may be influenced by many factors, one of the most important being the desire for change. The first step by the staff should be to learn as much as possible about the participants' backgrounds and special interests.

Participants have experiences that can be shared and on which activities can be based. They may have had capabilities that they can no longer utilize because of dysfunction, but their interests can provide a starting point for participation. Some motivating factors may be

- a desire to please others and the need for approval
- an association between a past pleasing experience and the task at hand
- the social rewards of sharing
- the intrinsic value of creativity and achievement
- curiosity as a learning incentive
- the recognition given by others
- a way to build competence.

The activity leader should act as a catalyst. Strictly speaking, one does not motivate others; motivation comes through self-actualization. An impetus to change may awaken dormant abilities. Getting a lawyer, longshoreman, or gardener interested in activities, possibly for the first time, may be as easy or as hard as getting to know them, and depends in large measure on how the activities are presented. Many will join in right from the start. But how will the withdrawn or the depressed be drawn in? It is not always easy. It will take time, tact, and sensitivity, but usually it can be done.

MOTIVATION METHODS

There are a few principles that will help ensure success. First, make the newcomer feel welcome. (Prior review of significant disabilities and careful accommodation to them will put the person at ease more quickly.) Staff members, wearing name tags, should greet each participant by name and should have determined before his or her arrival whether, for example, the person should stay in a wheelchair or can safely walk in the reception room.

Allow time to talk to the newcomers individually to discuss their reasons for attending, their interests, and their abilities. Explain the program to them and encourage questions. Introduce the new arrivals to the other participants, particularly those who have similar interests; they can play an important role in welcoming the newcomers and helping to relieve the tension and any feelings of being outsiders.

Treat the participants as the adults they are. Assume that they have led full lives and have extensive knowledge, dignity, and a sense of humor. They deserve respect and will respond to it. Whatever activities are presented, they should have appeal for adults and there should be some range of choice.

Offer activities based on goals determined by and shared with the participants, suited to their needs and interests, that can be done as independently as possible.

In the beginning, select activities in which the participants can experience success. Many have suffered a loss of self-esteem and need to regain mastery of something, no matter how small. Participants should be made to feel that what they are doing is appreciated by someone else. This calls for credit when it is due—not flattery. A compliment on something that obviously did not turn out well is belittling; but recognition of whatever advances were made in the process, however slight, is rewarding.

Allow for continuing staff-participant interaction to ensure that needs and goals are being met.

Allow for changes in the participants' abilities through variety and a range of activities, keeping in mind the various ethnic, religious, educational, age, and other characteristics of the participants.

PROBLEMS IN MOTIVATING

It may be difficult, if not impossible, to involve some individuals. In these instances, the staff may feel a sense of failure. Some participants have a need to be alone at times, and this may make the staff uneasy. Forcing involvement may only increase a participant's anger or depression. Assuring the person that it is all right to be a spectator (allowing a choice) is often a good approach toward encouraging interest. Someone who always withdraws into isolation may need more stimulus. Sometimes, asking a question that cannot be answered by "No" helps. Instead of asking, "Would you like to do this?" it may be better to ask, "Which one would you like to work on?"

Everything is not going to be successful for everyone. The participant whose only motivation to come to the program is to please a family member will probably not demonstrate any enthusiasm. The lifetime loner may never join in by choice. The totally disoriented person may not be capable of participation. Even those who meet none of the physical or cognitive goals set by the staff may derive some psychosocial benefits by opportunities to be in touch with the outside world. Social and emotional support in itself can be a reason for continuing.

Time is sometimes critical. We all travel at our own pace and readiness for involvement will differ. Someone who has been housebound or isolated for years will require more nurturing than one who comes in straight from a rehabilitation hospital. A person who has suffered a recent loss of function may need more time to accept and adjust to the loss. It is important to move slowly in directing the interest of the reluctant participant. A person may voluntarily join in a group game one day, after seemingly unending encouragement, then pull back into a shell when scheduled for, say, three hours of card playing the next session.

Those who have communication problems may require special help. A speech therapist (if available) may be able to suggest ways in which the staff can encourage better speech or communication. Some people with speech deficits may comprehend perfectly what is being said, without being able to communicate. Others may have comprehension problems as well, and require special types of instruction (e.g., structured, step-by-step demonstrations given separately from verbal direction). Communication aids, such as alphabet boards, writing or typing, the use of globes, pictures, maps, or magazines may be of assistance in helping such persons to be a part of the group.

Each staff member should attempt to develop sensitivity to the participants' emotional and physical stress. This is called empathy—putting oneself into others' shoes, in an attempt to understand what they are experiencing. This does not mean sympathizing; it means recognizing their feelings and helping them cope with them. It is often necessary to give attention to these needs first. Distracting the participants by putting them immediately into an activity does not help the situation. A little time spent in listening and perhaps sharing the pain may be the therapy needed for the moment.

Participants' difficulties in approaching their own goals may be unwittingly frustrated by others (e.g., the staff member who corrects or redoes a project, the family member who belittles an accomplishment, or the well-meaning friend who shows what the participant used to be able to do). Education of a participant's roommate, spouse, and friends should be part of the program for someone who lacks self-assurance.

Learning to let go of participants may be difficult for some staff members. Those who have achieved a measure of independence must be allowed to use it and expand it in other fields. Attempting to assist someone who no longer requires help only encourages dependency. Value must be placed on the person's own accomplishments. This does not mean they can be ignored. They will always need encouragement and recognition.

Chapter 4

Operating the Program

The therapeutic activities program is usually coordinated by a registered occupational therapist working with a team of aides, assistants, and volunteers. In some institutions, a trained recreation therapist may be the leader. The team members usually come from widely differing backgrounds and fields of experience. Therefore, it is essential that each team member be willing to surrender some professional autonomy so that the group can work smoothly. Genuine teamwork precludes concern with professional jurisdiction. As the team members become more and more involved in the program, they often display capabilities that they may not have realized they had. Like the participants, they often find that they enjoy working in parts of the program they had previously considered uninteresting. In one instance, a woman who had been a barber discovered that she had a talent for teaching woodworking, something she had never done before. As the efforts of team members blend, they discover a feeling of freedom in carrying out their various roles in a more creative manner.

KEYS TO EFFECTIVENESS

Some important elements in an effective activities program are: a simple, well-defined structure that is treatment-goal oriented, flexibility, in-service education, and continuous communication.

Structure helps to keep the program from being caught up in business that might obscure the underlying therapeutic goals. For a moment, visualize a therapeutic activities program for disabled elderly. There are several large, pleasant rooms with a great deal going on and everyone apparently engrossed in what is happening.

TYPICAL ACTIVITIES

It is November, and much of the work is on projects for the annual Christmas boutique. Last year's proceeds from the participants' handcrafts netted over $1,200, and the members voted to use the money for craft equipment, supplies, and some pots and pans for the training kitchen. The year before, the proceeds were used to buy a piano.

An elderly, arthritic woman has completed an eyeglasses case for the sale. "They're going to ask five dollars for it," she announces with some pride. Now she can return to her red-white-and-blue Bargello pillow. She will be taking it home with her when it is finished, and with it a new skill, something aesthetically satisfying.

Six men and women, half of them in wheelchairs, are at an oblong table supervised by the art instructor. Most of them are working on marketable Christmas wreaths, dipping small pine cones and berries into white glue and sticking them to circular cardboard frames. The activity has a therapeutic value for the participants, some of whom have suffered strokes. Reaching for the glue pot may increase range of motion; sorting out pine cones and inserting them into the design may improve perception and help with fine muscle control. Producing something of quality will almost certainly increase the sense of self-esteem and bring a feeling of fulfillment.

Another woman finishes a wreath, which goes on the rack for the sale items, and then moves to the center of the room. It is easy to mistake her for a member of the staff. She has no problem in walking, no speech problem, and apparent use of all her faculties. But a year ago she had a serious heart attack. She was 50 pounds heavier at that time, but, with encouragement from her fellow participants, she has lost this extra weight and is now attractively slender. With help from the nutritionist, she has learned how to prepare foods for her diet in the adjoining kitchen. She will soon be leaving the program as a formal participant, but has expressed a wish to return as a volunteer.

Her main problem, not immediately observable, is lack of confidence. The occupational therapy assistant has set up a board for her, with brass nails tacked in a numbered pattern, around which she is to wind colored strings for a wall hanging of string art. "You have more confidence in me than I have," she says to the assistant. That is true, but, it is also true that her confidence is growing. A few months earlier, she would not even try something new. Now, however, she reads the directions, takes a deep breath, and says, "Well, I guess a woman who has raised seven children ought to be able to do this." And she does it.

Another participant looks alert and well, until he tries to speak; coordinated movement appears difficult for him. He has Parkinson's disease, which impairs his ability to move freely and affects his speech musculature. His activities are aimed at helping him to utilize his abilities through special muscle exercise. After a few minutes of pushing a weighted box equipped with handles up and down a slanted board—a task designed to maintain his strength and keep him mobile—he goes into the solarium to join in other activities. The verbal interaction that will go on at this game is designed to reinforce the speech therapy he gets regularly. With the exception of the staff member, none of the card players speaks clearly, but they are encouraged to talk during the game. If they succeed in recovering even enough speech to make their basic needs known, their life at home will be somewhat easier.

One of the card players can use only one hand since his stroke. But other participants have made small slotted wooden stands to hold cards, so now he can stand his cards up while drawing new ones or waiting his turn to play. The purpose of the game is to match cards to take a trick. Nothing is hurried. There are no concessions because someone is confused, as one of the players discovers. The player with the card holder helps the confused one and there is tacit agreement among the group that such help is fair. Regardless of the disability, the best player wins.

After 30 minutes of cards, the players go back to the large activities room. There is a soft hum of activity. A former commercial artist who has lost the use of one hand is sketching another participant. In the protective atmosphere of the activities program he again has an opportunity to use his skill. This provides him with an emotional outlet and adds to his self-esteem and confidence. His sketches are displayed on bulletin boards around the room, as are examples of other people's drawings, string art, weaving, posters—all products of the regulated, scheduled activity.

Without the system, which includes profiles of each participant's daily efforts and a chart of scheduled activities for each one's day, there could be disorganization, with neglected, overlooked people working aimlessly. The participants' charts, the staff's knowledge of each individual problem, and the treatment goals provide a sense of direction and continuity as each person moves through the program. The atmosphere is pervaded with a sense of purpose and control, which provides comfort and protection for the participants. One member said, "Here, everyone cares. I feel so free and yet so safe."

PROGRAM STRUCTURE

Although the program's activities are based on the participants' needs and interests, the participants do not control the program. If they did, many of them would pursue projects they found easy and pleasant, rather than working on tasks that include the therapeutic activities they need. Others would proceed aimlessly, finding it difficult to choose a project or to persevere in working on one. Structure is especially important for such people, and for those who are easily distracted.

Most participants feel safer in a clearly defined setting with gentle, firm direction rather than in a very active, busy environment where they are left to themselves.

Structure also makes possible continuous monitoring of the participants. The monitoring plan is essentially a carefully thought-out treatment plan. It provides the staff with a clear, well-defined set of goals for each person, with simple forms to keep regular records on how the goals are being met. This makes it possible to adjust each program as needed.

Structure also implies careful, detailed scheduling of time and space. The initial analysis of the goals for each participant often reveals clusters of people with similar needs who can be grouped together for particular kinds of activities, such as discussion groups (for intellectual or speech stimulation) or handcrafts aimed at specific goals.

But structure need not imply rigidity. The activities program needs a balance between structure and flexibility, especially where some of the participants attend part-time, where some of the staff are also part-time employees, and where most of the volunteers are able to serve only one or two days a week. The emphasis in a therapeutic activities program is usually on those elements that are imaginative and innovative, and this calls for staff members and volunteers with a wide variety of talents, interests, and skills. It is usually exceedingly difficult to recruit full-time staff who can bring to the program the richness that will make it truly therapeutic. This is because of budget limitations and the fact that many persons interested in the program may not be able to work full time. It seems best, then, to divide the funds budgeted for full-time staff among several part-time staff members, depending upon the number of people expected to participate in the program. These decisions will vary with local conditions.

The flexibility provided by a part-time staff with a wide range of skills and experience is offset by scheduling problems, but with adequate supervision the benefits far outweigh the inconveniences. For this flexibility in use of staff to work, however, there must be a full-time staff person in charge. As noted earlier, the coordinator is often an occupational therapist. This seems to work quite effectively, because this kind of therapist usually has the professional training and experience needed to supervise the program. The occupational therapist can oversee the total program and make certain that the goals are translated into day-to-day activities.

EDUCATION FOR STAFF

A permanent in-service education program is another key part of the therapeutic activities program. New staff members need to learn about the various disabilities of the participants and the effect of those conditions on behavior. They must be able to recognize signs of fatigue or stress and how to deal with them. They need to know that sometimes behavior that may be irritating and frustrating to them and to other participants may often be a residual effect of a disability. They need to learn the techniques of transferring people into and out of wheelchairs, how to lock them safely, how to push the wheelchairs over doorsills, and, where necessary, how to move wheelchairs safely into and out of elevators. In addition, they should learn other crafts besides those in which they specialize. It is the responsibility of the occupational therapist coordinating the program to see that the in-service education is an integral part of the overall program.

The coordinator must also monitor the activities program to make certain that the treatment goals for individuals are respected. For example, an arthritic participant may complain about working on a project at an elevated level or angle. Trying to be helpful, a staff aide might then permit the participant to lower the level or reduce the angle, thereby reducing the therapeutic value of the activity. The coordinator can state the reason for not modifying what the participant is doing in such a way that the aide is not embarrassed but learns something about how to handle the patient. Another example of what can happen is that staff members, feeling sorry for blind participants, feed them instead of helping them feed themselves. Here, again, a good supervisor can preserve the staff member's relationship with the participant while explaining the significance of the activity for developing independence. Regular supervision and in-service education can reduce such errors and increase the program's effectiveness.

Weekly staff meetings centered around individual participants' needs and goals help to keep the staff functioning as a team. The regular, formalized interaction of staff meetings can also be used to encourage informal staff learning. The sharing of books and articles is a usual practice. Staff are also encouraged to take courses and broaden knowledge. But perhaps the most effective on-the-job education occurs through free and open communication among the staff. When all the staff members intermingle in the various program activities throughout the day, changes in participant behavior and any problems that arise can be observed and dealt with. Techniques for handling problems and problem behavior can be seen in operation. Staff-participant interaction can also be observed and later, in staff sessions, can be evaluated with respect to the overall program goals.

The rapport that flows out of good communication also fosters another kind of flexibility, namely, movement of staff members within various parts of the program. A volunteer came to one facility expecting to help with speech therapy, but discovered that she simply could not do it. A shift to another program element, working with handcrafts, helped her to feel more comfortable and enabled her to contribute to the program in a way that gave her a sense of fulfillment. In another instance, administrative flexibility made possible the assignment of a craft instructor to those crafts she liked best and knew the most about, and her obvious enthusiasm carried over to the participants and they benefited from her instruction.

Chapter 5

The Use of Volunteers

Professional staff leadership is essential to the program, but the use of volunteer staff members is equally important for diversification and program enrichment. Volunteerism is often erroneously equated with non-professionalism. Volunteers are people endowed with the entire range of abilities and experiences found within the general population from which the paid staff comes. They must be respected for the special abilities, experience, and motivation they bring to the program. Volunteers must never supplant the paid staff, but should augment it. Volunteers can expand the professional services that institutions are able to provide with paid staff.

In addition to supplying program skills and staff-support functions, volunteers also perform an important community-relations service. Their awareness of the contributions that a program makes to its participants enables them to become effective interpreters of the program in the community. They are often able to recruit others to fill volunteer roles, and may be willing to seek other types of community support for the program.

There are also psychodynamic aspects of the role of the volunteer who provides direct service to the handicapped. It may be that a person who is ill or handicapped experiences a change in body image or mental function, and there can be a need for renewal of identity. The volunteer, by representing an intact identity, can serve as a role model for the handicapped person. As the participant begins to move toward increased community participation, the volunteer becomes increasingly important as a model for health. Often participants have experienced some degree of isolation and need help to reestablish normal interpersonal functioning. The volunteer who is sensitive to the participants' needs is often the staff person who can devote additional time to a participant in need of attention.

RECRUITMENT AND MOTIVATION

Properly recruited, trained, and supervised, volunteers can contribute greatly to the activities program. Before any recuiting is done, the program administrator should develop an inventory of possible volunteer positions, including program consultants, activity aides, community-relations experts, and indirect-service functionaries.

Volunteer consultants can provide guidance to the paid staff in program development. A professional photographer, artist, sculptor, graphics designer, home economist, or crafts specialist who is not interested in volunteering on a regular basis might be willing to guide the staff in program design or to advise the administrator of other human or physical resources. A one-time demonstration of a particular craft would be another likely contribution.

These program activity aides would work directly under a paid staff member in a specific activity—e.g., needlework, clay, or string art, and an aide who is highly skilled in a particular craft might even be the activity leader. However, a paid staff member should be assigned to work with the volunteer leader to assure program continuity.

Volunteers can perform community-relations functions such as seeking scrap materials and other donations from organizations and commercial sources, recruiting other volunteers, providing interagency liaison activities, etc. They can also help with indirect-service functions such as clerical duties, general program work, recording, mailing, duplicating, collating, handling inventory and supplies, etc.

Requirements for specific jobs should be determined by the administrator in consultation with the paid staff and be based on the needs and interests of the participants. If there is a keen interest in a group newspaper, for example, and no one is able to provide the necessary leadership, this might be one of the volunteer positions for which candidates would be recruited.

Most communities are filled with excellent sources of volunteer help and with motivated volunteers. The challenge is to tap every possible source, to interpret the volunteer opportunity effectively, and then to make it attractive for the recruit. Volunteers may be recruited from local service organizations, service clubs, colleges, newcomers clubs, councils for the arts, and employee service groups in large corporations. Newspapers and senior citizen newsletters may be willing to run feature articles describing the program and its opportunities for volunteers. Once a nucleus of volunteers has been formed and program responsibilities are well defined, the recruitment effort will be enhanced by their spreading the word about their experiences. Volunteer service can add meaning to the lives of all people. It provides a chance for them to give to society, rather than just receive, and can enhance self-identity and self-esteem.

People volunteer for many reasons, including the following:

- productive use of skills and time
- opportunities for training and for pre-vocational sampling
- expectation of social contacts in a new community
- opportunity to care for others
- diversional activity for self-help purposes.

SELECTION AND ORIENTATION

Understanding the volunteer's motivation is an important part of the selection process. Not everyone who offers makes a good volunteer, but the interviewer should make every initial interview a constructive experience and should recommend other avenues to pursue if the volunteer is unsuitable. The needs of the volunteer may conflict with the purpose, functions, and goals of the program, and this conflict may not be apparent until after the volunteer has become involved. But carefully planned orientation usually allows sufficient time to evaluate the new volunteer.

Part of the application process for volunteers should include a skills inventory and self-evaluation checklist which will enable them to explain their special interests, likes, and dislikes. During the selection interview, the specific assignment being considered and the time it will take must be clearly stated. Detailed job descriptions are helpful for all concerned. Volunteers should learn something about the history and goals of the program, as well as some of the psychological, physical, and social characteristics of the groups being served. They should be encouraged to reveal their reactions to the setting, proposed assignments, and their own expectations and aims.

Willingness to serve and an interest in handicapped individuals do not by themselves make a person an effective volunteer. Effectiveness in working with people and an ability to relate personally but remain objective in relationships with all the members of the group are essential. Following careful screening and the appropriate assignment, a volunteer should be asked to serve for a stated job-orientation trial period.

The staff supervisor is responsible for making the volunteer's experience a satisfying and useful one. However, if it does not prove to be a successful assignment or if the volunteer has problems in relating to the participants, the time-limited orientation makes termination less difficult for the volunteer. Volunteers who have problems must be given the benefit of staff analysis of the situation and an opportunity to sample other assignments. Some may find that they do not enjoy working directly with the participants but can carry out indirect-service assignments. The investment of staff time in the selection and orientation process will be well repaid through the advantage of having carefully placed, satisfied volunteers and an enriched program.

Orientation is usually done individually, but a training workshop for volunteers should also be scheduled. Volunteers are usually recruited one at a time and lose interest if they are not given immediate placement. To help orient the volunteer before the formal training workshop and to reinforce the many new pieces of information given orally, it is useful to have a manual that briefly describes the facility and program, administrative routines, record keeping, and responsibilities of the volunteer.

TRAINING

There should be a plan for training and supervision, once the volunteer has been oriented and permanently assigned to a job. The staff supervisor should design a training plan with the volunteer, including an opportunity for periodic conferences during which the volunteer can talk about findings, problems, and suggestions. Training may include attendance at skills workshops in the community, observation of other parts of the facility program, attendance at in-service education programs designed for the paid staff, and sharing of instructional materials. Volunteers identify with the program and its goals if they are included in staff meetings and if they are asked to give their evaluations of participants' progress. A volunteer who has capabilities pertinent to the program might be invited to conduct a training session for other staff members.

ASSIGNMENT

A volunteer's special abilities should be utilized on the job unless the volunteer has specifically asked that it be otherwise. Sometimes a volunteer seeks an opportunity to develop new capabilities or may want a change from a well-performed task. The availability of a volunteer sometimes permits the program coordinator to add features that could not be afforded through assignment of paid staff. In some cases, these activities may not be directly related to the existing crafts program, but provide needed socialization and educational opportunities for the participants.

Examples of such activities are the following:

- Friendly visiting with participants as they arrive in the morning, over a cup of coffee or juice, at lunch, or while awaiting transportation at the end of the day.

- A concerned volunteer with a good sense of humor and ability to listen can provide valuable personal contacts.
- Table games, including card games. These games are popular, and a volunteer can teach new ones. Participants vary in ability, but the volunteer staff member can assist in forming compatible groups.
- Horseshoes, bean bag or ball throwing, and table shuffleboard are other examples of competitive games for small groups that cannot be offered when the number of participants is large and the paid staff is small. Games that emphasize chance and do not depend on physical skill are more popular.
- Current events discussion groups.
- Travel lectures using slides or movies not exceeding 20 minutes in duration.
- Cooking for fun.
- Horticulture programs, such as windowsill gardening, or outdoor projects when weather permits.
- Music programs.

These are supplementary to the many craft activities discussed in this volume and permit a change of pace for participants in an all-day program. As volunteers become acquainted with participants, they learn more of their interests and can undoubtedly produce suggestions for ways to improve the program.

With adequate orientation, appropriate assignments, continuing supervision, and training opportunities, the volunteer program should be successful. Depending on the number of volunteers and the size of the entire program, it may be necessary for the administrator to designate one staff member as coordinator of volunteers. This person would be responsible for such matters as annual recognition of volunteers, handling minor day-to-day problems, and providing a channel of communication between the program administrator and the volunteers.

POTENTIAL PROBLEMS

Some possible problems for inexperienced volunteers, and suggested remedies, are:

1. A volunteer who has a strong need to control and manage.

    - Define the assisting role precisely and make it clear at the outset that the volunteer is to be responsible to a particular staff member.

- Explain the reasons for the volunteer's assisting role and its relation to institutional policies, continuity of participants' care, and staff responsibilities.
- If the volunteer is unsatisfied with working under a particular staff member, explore the reason. (The volunteer may or may not need to be given another assignment.)

2. A volunteer who does not allow participants to function independently.

- Make clear to the volunteer the importance of independent functioning for participants. The goals should be defined in unambiguous terms to ensure understanding.
- If the problem continues, the volunteer's motivation should be examined. If the volunteer is to be retained, transfer to a non-client assignment may be better, along with an explanation of the need for assistance in another function, either within or outside the department.

3. A volunteer who is inconsistent in attendance.

- If the service is truly needed, obtain a commitment on the amount of time and number of days the volunteer can attend. (Most volunteers who feel their services are useful to the facility will be reliable. It should be understood, however, that volunteers cannot be expected to give as much of their time as paid staff members do.)
- If the volunteer consistently changes attendance time or cancels, determine the reason. If the volunteer's personal life does not allow for regular attendance, consider transfer to a non-client-related project that can be done with little staff supervision and maximum flexibility as to time.
- If assignments cannot be adjusted or the volunteer cannot accept a new schedule, explain the need for regular attendance and discontinue the arrangement until a time when a more reliable commitment can be made.

4. A volunteer who befriends a participant, to the detriment of the program. (This may result in problems for other members of the group who resent the extra attention given to one member. It can create problems for the staff and interfere with treatment. It can also become difficult for the volunteer, because the participant can manipulate the relationship and make demands the volunteer is unable to meet.)

- Discuss the problem with the participant and offer an opportunity to modify the relationship by working with another volunteer who can be alerted to the problem.
- Give the volunteer an opportunity to discuss the problem in a non-threatening atmosphere so as to uncover the reason for the behavior.
- Give the volunteer an opportunity for greater involvement with the other participants.

5. A volunteer who after a period of service is physically or mentally incapable of continuing. This may develop at any time, and steps should be taken to remove or reassign the volunteer. Often the volunteer recognizes the problem and may be relieved to be able to discontinue service in a tactful, face-saving manner.
6. A volunteer who wastes staff time. Some volunteers see the program as an avenue for education. If they can learn by participation while contributing where the need exists, this can work well for both the volunteer and the staff. However, if the volunteer expects instruction beyond the needs of the assignment or demands information relating to participants beyond that needed for working effectively, the staff could be spending an inappropriate amount of time with the volunteer, to the neglect of participants. Some volunteers work for only a short time because of service requirements for an organization or required school credits and have little motivation to be of assistance beyond fulfilling the time requirement. Clearly, the effort involved in orientating these volunteers is poorly spent. This problem can be avoided through careful screening in the initial interview. If a person in this situation slips through screening, gentle confrontation with frank, open discussion is in order.

The successful integration of volunteers and paid staff in the activities program is beneficial for the staff and participants alike. The administrator who has a commitment to, and conviction about, the value of volunteers is usually willing to make the necessary investment of time and effort needed to assure its success.

Chapter 6

The Facility

An activities program can be operated in any one of a variety of settings. The most important consideration in the choice and use of a facility is the psychological influence of the environment. It is a well-documented fact that loud contrasting colors can act as a stimulant, and that cool tones can provide a calming influence. Music that is loud and of rapid tempo can be unpleasantly stimulating. Many persons who have suffered loss or trauma require structure in their lives and an environment that provides ease and tranquillity.

IMPORTANT FACTORS

Some of the crucial questions to be considered in creating such an environment are:

- What is the building's accessibility? Is it a major task for participants just to get into it?
- Is there space to maneuver inside? (Having to move every time another person enters or leaves a room can be quite distracting.)
- Do the colors of the walls, ceilings, floor coverings, and furnishings blend harmoniously?
- How is the wall space used? Is every inch of space covered with tools, equipment, and projects? (If so, this may produce a feeling of being closed in.)
- Is there a sense of organization, giving the participant a feeling of being expected, or are the materials piled and scattered about without any seeming order?

- Is the facility arranged so as to foster socialization, or do the work spaces face walls and thus encourage isolated activity?
- Does the facility have a quiet place for those who need occasional rest or privacy?
- Is the arrangement conducive to self-help, or are things organized in such a way as to encourage dependence?
- Are staff members available to help if needed?
- If the facility is small, have efforts been made to remove unnecessary furnishings or displays?
- Do participants have an opportunity to influence the environment?

With many programs, the assigned space may not be ideal and adaptations may be needed to make it more convenient for the disabled. Architectural barriers such as stairs can often be made more accessible with ramps. A room can be used for several programs; dividers may allow more flexibility. The proper use of space depends on the size of the supervising staff and the type and number of participants. With a small staff, supervision and coordination of activities is easiest in one area so the staff can assist one another more easily. If the program encompasses more staff members, with different concurrent activities, groups can be separated for a more effective program. For example:

- A structured-game group with confused or disoriented participants is best housed in a small, quiet room where distractions can be kept to a minimum.
- A music program may need more space, if instruments are involved, and separation from a craft area where verbal instructions are being given.
- Woodworking should be done in a closed, well-ventilated room because of the noise and dust it generates.

The proper selection and use of furnishings and equipment is important in making the facility more functional.

FLOORS

Floors should be kept uncarpeted for easier wheelchair management, housekeeping, and maintenance (with spillage, etc.). Surfaces must be non-slip (avoid heavy wax). A solid color floor is better than a patterned one for those with visual or perceptual problems. If there are any places where the floor level changes (e.g., the entry to a bathroom), it should be leveled off by removal of aprons. If the difference in level cannot be eliminated, a brightly colored tape or paint can be applied where the level change occurs to alert participants to the danger.

DOORS

Doors must allow for easy opening; avoid strong door springs. The opening must be wide enough to allow for wheelchair clearance (32 inches minimum clear width when the door is opened at 90 degrees).

WINDOWS

It is ideal to have an outdoor view from activity rooms so that participants can observe changes in nature. Lined draperies may be advisable for rooms used to show movies. Local fire regulations should be checked regarding requirements for window hangings. Some sun worshippers prefer sitting close to windows; others, such as those with cataracts, may find direct sunlight visually irritating. Those with certain neurological diseases, such as multiple sclerosis, may become fatigued by too much direct sunlight.

TABLES

The most important factors in selection of work tables are stability and accessibility. Small craft groups where participants are doing a variety of activities generally work best at round tables because the staff can get around more easily to provide individual attention, and opportunities for social interaction are increased. Oblong tables are best for group projects where supplies and equipment require more space. Small square tables are more suitable for board or card games, because reaching is easier. It is best to avoid tables with aprons, which limit leg room and make it difficult to attach vises. Narrow tables are also difficult for wheelchair users because of inadequate leg clearance.

Participants and staff members must be able to get around tables easily, so table placement is crucial. When craft tables are also used for food service or trays, round tables are inconvenient. Pedestal tables have good leg clearance but are usually not as stable. (Participants must be cautioned not to use them for support when standing up.) Tables in a woodworking room should be heavy (a hard wood such as maple is preferred) to withstand pounding.

CHAIRS

Good support is a crucial factor in the selection of chairs. They should have full arms and should preferably be padded on the back and seat and covered with a sturdy washable material. The chairs should be of standard height (18 inches), with straight seats and backs for easier, safer transfers to and from wheelchairs.

VENTILATION

Cross ventilation is preferred. The temperature should be controllable if possible. Most older people require more warmth in the winter than young people, but are more easily fatigued by hot weather. Air conditioning, if not well controlled, may prove too cold for the older person. Protected outdoor spaces can be utilized on temperate days for certain activities.

STORAGE UNITS

If space is ample storage units should be built in to give more flexibility in the use of wall space. However, built-in units in small rooms reduce the space available for activities and can be inconvenient if the nature of the program changes.

Five types of storage that have proved successful are:

1. open closets with low racks for hanging coats
2. wide shelved closets with sliding doors and sliding racks for hanging of bagged items and deep storage for large equipment (e.g., table looms)
3. locked fireproof cabinets for storage of flammable supplies and expensive equipment
4. open-rack shelving for drying and storage of individual projects
5. wall pegboards for craft display and hanging of tools and large frames

An important objective in choice of storage is accessibility. Frequently used tools, equipment, and work in process should be stored at a level where the participants can reach them.

Storage organization is covered in Chapter 7, Equipment and Supplies.

BATHROOMS

Bathrooms should be close to activity rooms and should permit easy access. (See *Bathroom Equipment*, Appendix A.) Grab rails are essential; they are inexpensive and easily installed. Toilet safety frames are attached directly to the toilet and require no wall supports. (See Appendix A.) Special equipment of this kind should be checked frequently to make certain it is functioning properly. There should be good clearance under the washbasins for wheelchair users, and wall mirrors should be low enough for easy viewing from a wheelchair.

Although electric hand dryers on walls have proved to be more sanitary and easier to use than hand towels for some wheelchair users, they tie up bathrooms for longer periods and, being mechanical, have occasional breakdowns. A good solution is accessible hand towels supplemented by electric hand dryers.

BASINS

Where there are under-basin cabinets, doors can be removed and top space cut out or a bottom shelf removed to make leg clearance for wheelchair users. Long-handled faucets are preferable to the knob type. (Knob faucets can be adapted. See Appendix A.) Suction-cup brushes (See Appendix A) should be at all washbasins to help one-handed participants to be independent in their clean-up.

It is difficult to conduct an innovative arts or crafts program without easy access to water, although it can be brought from another room if necessary. If possible, sinks used for craft activities should be of the chemical laboratory type to reduce chronic drain clogging.

USEFUL ITEMS

A bulletin board is convenient for posting schedules and providing space for participants and staff to post items of news or special interest. It should be in a central place where people can wheel or walk to it and should be easily visible.

A public telephone is almost a necessity in a large facility. It should be open and low enough to permit use from a wheelchair.

If a television set is available, it should be mounted high enough for all to see it easily. A remote control switch will enable the staff to control its use.

NOTE

Helpful information on adapting activity space in a facility can be found in American National Standard Specifications for Making Buildings and Facilities Accessible to, and Usable by, Physically Handicapped People, Document Number A 117. 1-1980. The information is available from the American National Standards Institute, 1430 Broadway, New York, NY 10018 (1980) for $5.00 plus $2.00 handling charge.

Chapter 7
Equipment and Supplies

The resources available and the need for equipment and supplies vary within each facility to such an extent that what seems basic for one program might be considered a luxury for another. The tools and equipment referred to throughout this manual have been selected to facilitate independence. (See Appendix B.) It is generally wise to invest in a minimum of supplies and equipment at the beginning, until there is some certainty about the nature of the participants and the skills of the staff. Expendable supplies need not be expensive, but it is wise to purchase good, reputable brands for the basic equipment.

USE OF DISCARDED MATERIALS

Scrap materials may be used for many projects. As one participant pointed out in a facility newsletter, "Your junk is our treasure." Both the staff and the participants soon begin to think of new ways to use almost any kind of container or material. This has therapeutic value in itself. Examples of things available in nearly every household that have proved useful in an activities program are:

- aluminum beverage cans
- aluminum trays
- cardboard tubes from rolls of waxed paper, aluminum foil, etc.
- crayons
- garden and seed catalogs
- jars and bottles
- plastic margarine containers

- old beads and jewelry
- old eyeglass lenses
- old greeting cards and pictures
- old sheets, wool, and other material
- picture calendars
- plastic pill boxes and bottles
- scrap pieces of wood, leather, vinyl, cloth, and yarn
- shoe boxes.

The challenge of collecting such usable materials can be taken on as an assignment by a women's club, scouting group, or other service organization. Scouts can also gather nature materials. Showing a group a finished product may help motivate them. Local merchants can be asked to help. Let a shoe-store operator know that shoe boxes are needed, or tell a grocer that the program could use tomato baskets. Ask to be called when a supply is available, and arrange to pick them up. Many supply companies will give discounts on materials for a non-profit organization upon presentation of a certificate showing tax-exempt status. Others will donate materials outright. A fabric company, for instance, may give a large quantity of discontinued material to an activities program, or a lumber company may donate wood.

EXPENSIVE ITEMS

When expensive materials are called for, it may be necessary to limit the number of projects a participant completes, or those who work rapidly may be asked to pay for the material if they choose to make more than one item. If kits are expensive, a solution may be to purchase one kit to use as a model for other units to be made from raw materials.

BORROWING

A community can also provide other activity resources. The public library might make a revolving loan of books, especially those in larger type, and a mobile library might agree to make the facility one of its regular stops. Schools and libraries have films and filmstrips that can be borrowed, and they may be willing to lend their projectors as well as records and record players.

SAFETY

Safety comes first in all activities. Dangerously heavy or high-speed electrical equipment generally should be limited to staff use. When hot wax is used, as in batik, the work must be carefully supervised and probably should be restricted to those who can feel heat and whose psychomotor coordination indicates the ability to use it safely.

Smoking should never be permitted in craft rooms, because of the paper, turpentine, paint rags, and other combustible materials being used. Also, smoking fumes are a major irritant and hazardous to the health of the participants. Fire regulations and insurance requirements must be adhered to and may limit the use of equipment and space.

Clamps and vises, which are convenient and often necessary, also contribute to safety in stabilizing equipment for those who are unable to hold work steady. However, they must be securely fastened to the table or bench.

Accessibility is essential in the storage of materials because a major goal of the activities program is to increase participant independence and to build self-confidence and self-esteem. A simple color-coding procedure is effective in organizing tools, equipment, and work in process.

ORGANIZATION OF EQUIPMENT AND SUPPLIES

Woodworking Room

Essential Items

1. pegboard and hooks
2. colored plastic tape
3. black felt-tip pens
4. shelves
5. wall space

Procedure

Arrange the tools on the pegboard with the proper hooks. Put a strip of colored tape around each tool and a piece of the same color tape on the pegboard above it. Put a number on the tape on each tool and the same number on the pegboard below it. An alternative method for tool storage is to cut out a contact-paper silhouette of the tool and mount it on the pegboard.

Tools and equipment that cannot hang handily on pegboards should be placed on shelves, following a procedure similar to the foregoing. Tape and number the tool, give it its own spot on the shelf, and place an identical tape and number on the edge of the shelf.

Rags, sandpaper, newspapers, etc., can be stored in deep boxes on shelves. The boxes should be numbered like the tools and should be returned to their places on the shelves following use.

Look for wall spaces other than the pegboard wall that can hold lightweight equipment (a long nail can hold yardsticks, T-squares, etc.). Participant safety should be kept constantly in mind when putting protruding nails in walls for hanging. Utilize every available space that will be handy to the staff and participants, color coding wherever possible.

When everything is in place, and the arranging and rearranging (and there will be some!) has been done, make a list of everything that is coded. This will be a checklist for the end of the day, and an instant inventory. Each storage unit should have such a list.

Craft Room

Essential Items

1. closets
2. shelves
3. wall space
4. colored plastic tape
5. black felt-tip pens
6. pegboard and hooks
7. bags with handles
8. sliding racks (such as used for trousers, ties, etc.)

Procedure

The procedure for color coding is the same as for the woodworking room. Mark the boxes, shelves, and tools in the same manner. If there are duplicate tools, color code for activity (e.g., yellow for woodworking, red for other crafts).

Boxes used to carry supplies such as thread, needles, scissors, and other sewing equipment from the shelves to the work tables each day can be covered in colorful contact paper before being taped and marked. Tomato boxes with handles (available from a grocer) are excellent for this; they are roomy and sturdy.

Shoe boxes, or larger boxes if needed, can be used to store participants' current projects on shelves or in closets. The name of the person should be printed on the box in large letters.

Sliding racks can be mounted in deep closets to hold each person's bag, arranged alphabetically by last name. These are particularly helpful with small yarn projects, such as needlework.

Tools for craft work can be hung on pegboard, as in the woodworking room. Paints stored by type are sufficiently visible so that only the shelves need be labeled to indicate their storage spots. Large paint brushes should be hung with bristles pointed down. Artists brushes, however, can be placed in jars or can holders, with the bristles up, and given a visible spot on a shelf.

Make a list, as for the woodworking room, and post it in a convenient spot for checking.

CAUTIONS

- The use of flammable supplies (such as turpentine and other thinners) must be carefully supervised by the staff and they must be returned to the flammable-storage cabinet immediately after use. A special metal container, with lid, is required for the disposal of rags and papers that have been used in working with varnish, stains, paints, thinners, etc.
- Garbage cans should be of the flip-top variety because they are easier to manipulate, particularly for those having the use of only one hand.
- Hand tools are generally preferable to electric tools for use by those with limited physical ability. (The use of any sharp tools by people with poor sensation or poor hand control should be carefully supervised.)
- Electrical equipment should be kept on a separate heavy table away from the participants' working area and its use should be closely supervised by the staff. It is preferable to have a staff member operate any power equipment.

SUMMARY

A color-coding system can be set up even with a small activities program. It makes checking on equipment and supplies at the day's end easier and faster, and there is less searching around for the required supplies the next day.

The visibility and accessibility of equipment and work in process encourages participants to pick out their own tools and work pieces instead of being "waited on." It encourages mobility and independence.

If the participants are involved in several diffcrent projects with different staff members, it is helpful to keep a record near each work space. Columns can be headed *Individual's Name, Project, Date Initiated,* and *Date Completed.* This information can be kept as a list or on a card system arranged alphabetically.

Chapter 8
A News Publication

Differences in interests, abilities, and backgrounds call for varied programs. It is advantageous to offer alternatives for participants who, for reasons of upbringing, physical limitations, or disinterest, do not enjoy or are unable to participate in an arts and crafts program. Some possibilities are horticulture (see Chapter 13), food preparation (see Chapter 9), organized games, and a news publication. Frequently, the last can supply a need for intellectual stimulation and promote therapeutic goals.

ESSENTIALS

A news publication can be as simple or as complex as the program can handle. It requires interested members who can share ideas and are capable of organization, as well as time, space, and equipment to produce it. A coordinating staff member is necessary for structuring, guidance, and continuity.

The opportunity for participants to make their own decisions on the nature of their publication is essential to success. Allowing them freedom to develop and expand the publication ensures their continuing interest.

Equipment and materials needed initially are simple: paper, a typewriter, and a means of duplicating the material. A stationery or paper company may be willing to donate or defray the cost of materials, and churches or other organizations are often willing to share duplicating equipment. Heavy stock is useful for a larger publication for the front and back, to make it more lasting for collectors and more adaptable to various cover-finishing techniques. Larger type helps for those who are more visually impaired.

The group members need not have literary skills. Some may be "idea people," serving as stimulators for others who have a greater knack for putting words together, and others may be more skilled in editing, typing, artwork, or production.

BENEFITS

A news publication can encourage increased awareness of one's environment (orientation), better organization of thought, increased self-expression, and improved social ability.

This kind of project provides people with group support and has the possibility of carry-over into the community and home.

SUCCESSFUL METHODS

Some guidelines for the staff in maintaining continuity and helping to stimulate the members are: Know the individuals' abilities and limitations. Be flexible about changes in group structure, allowing for different abilities and personality needs. Be open to new members joining the group, allowing them opportunities to participate or, if they desire, to withdraw comfortably. Allow the participants to contribute as they are able (e.g., some may be content to discuss, primarily, and do little actual writing). If nonverbal members are in the group, give them a chance to contribute. Through pictures, maps, or magazines, they may be able to express an idea for the group to work on, or they may be important on the production line. Allow those who are limited in physical abilities to contribute, even if they are unable to write (by dictating stories, poems, or jokes to another member, or using a tape machine to record ideas).

The publication can begin as a one-page chronicle of current happenings or a medium for creative writings, crossword puzzles, jokes, recipes, garden tips, etc. Participants may elect to have a theme for an issue, collecting and coordinating material of interest. The theme may go beyond the current knowledge of the group members, stimulating research (into community resources for the handicapped, for example).

The number of members on the team can vary, but eight to ten usually make up a stimulating but manageable group. How extensive such a publication should be will depend on the consistency of the group, how often they meet, and the resources available.

The members may elect to design a cover. A simple line drawing done by a participant can be enhanced by magic-marker coloring and duplicated, or a silk screening or block print can be used. Photography can be used if knowledge, equipment, and space are available.

Members can do the actual duplicating if the equipment is accessible to them. Assembly of the paper is a good team project and useful particularly for those who need activities to improve their organizational abilities.

The amount of staff coordination needed for such a project depends on the size of the participating group. There may be more than one group meeting at a time on the same issue. It is useful to have more than one staff member involved for continuity, in case one staff member is absent, and for the added capabilities and differing viewpoint. It is essential, however, that staff members agree on basic policies and meet regularly to coordinate their efforts.

One of the lasting rewards of paper publication can be increased self-esteem for participants. The publication should be distributed to families, friends, and the other participants in the facility. It gives visible recognition to those who may have limited skills in other fields.

The key to the use of this program is creativity. The publication that offers little more than duplication of previously printed material offers little incentive for developing ideas. The selection of a name for the publication, developing themes, and expressing individual and group ideas are effective sources of stimulation. The prime element in making it a successful and lasting project is in keeping it participant-centered.

Chapter 9

Food Preparation by Participants

The kitchen is often the center of activity in a household, and cooking, a necessary occupation, is often shared by men and women at some point in their lifetimes. Therefore, food preparation fits well into an activities program.

TASKS AND ABILITIES

The abilities required for food preparation are diverse and can be analyzed muscle by muscle. The physical abilities include reaching, pulling, pushing, lifting, carrying, holding, pinching, feeling, and seeing. Preparing a simple sandwich may involve opening a refrigerator door, opening a can, mixing, cutting, spreading, reaching for utensils and serving dishes, and carrying or transferring things to a table—all of which require physical and mental efforts in organizing, initiating, and carrying through a task.

An extensive cooking program may not be feasible without a kitchen. But with a hot plate, a few saucepans, mixing bowls, and basic utensils, simple dishes such as soup, popcorn, unbaked cookies, hors d'oeuvres, and salads can be prepared.

In this activity, as in others, people's abilities and interests vary. It cannot be assumed that someone with no previous interest in cooking will not participate. Even someone who has never been taught how to cook, and might be overwhelmed by attempting such an effort alone, can develop confidence through group sharing of tasks. Some people, because of changes at home, may no longer have the opportunity to do what was once a satisfying activity. Some people need to develop abilities for more active participation in matters at home.

Homemaking training for those returning to full responsibilities in the household can best be done by a trained therapist, but practice in skills and confidence building can be accomplished nicely in a group. The ideal group size depends on the work space and the amount of supervision required. For a group of multi-handicapped persons to prepare a lunch for themselves, involving two or more dishes, four or five persons usually work well together. Those who are ambulatory can handle activities at the counter level, and those who must remain seated can do things at the table, such as mixing and chopping.

Cooking is appropriate for most disability groups. People with severe brain damage or major problems in coordination should not attempt activities that require working with a stove or sharp instruments, but can, however, perform simple tasks such as kneading dough. Some persons who are too limited physically to participate in an activity might be included in helping to plan it. Precautions should be taken to safeguard those participants who have visual, sensory, or perceptual deficits.

GOALS

The therapeutic goals of cooking include the following:

- to assist people to become more independent and use their residual skills
- to help people maintain upper extremity function through activities such as reaching, opening, chopping, stirring, mixing, and kneading.
- to encourage greater tolerance for standing and for ambulatory activities through built-in mobility tasks (moving items from the stove to the refrigerator, sink, table, etc.)
- to reinforce a person's adherence to a diet by providing the opportunity to prepare tasty food that is within the diet limitations
- to help a person follow simple directions (e.g., reading recipes, following package directions, and following visual demonstrations)
- to rekindle interest in previously acquired abilities and experiences (if not limited by their diets, a group can try someone's favorite recipe)
- to facilitate the learning of new techniques as a stimulus (e.g., a different kind of cooking might be introduced, such as Chinese, which would be suitable for diabetics or those who must have a low calorie meal)
- to develop an awareness of the need for safety precautions, such as the use of barbecue mitts; the proper use of knives; the importance of good body positioning in relation to the activity at hand; the utilization of sliding racks, such as are found in the oven, to eliminate over-reaching; precautions in the use of burners, such as not leaning over them; and working from a person's best side

- to develop techniques in work simplification, such as better organization to reduce the number of steps involved, introducing short cuts by simplifying recipes, and using pre-chopped vegetables and one-dish meals
- to provide an opportunity for people to relate effectively to others and to share interests in a relaxed social atmosphere.

The time available may limit the tasks that can be undertaken in food preparation. Most people benefit from seeing an activity through from beginning to end. If necessary, participants who come to the facility daily can prepare a dish (such as a stew) one day and cook it the next day if time is limited.

CHOICES

Some possibilities for group cooking are:

- Preparing lunches, snacks, party fare, and desserts are particularly good activities. Others can share the food or those who prepare it can be encouraged to take the finished dishes home for family members, thus encouraging carry-over of the activity into the home. If food is prepared for a special holiday or occasion, those not involved in the cooking can help in planning the meal, setting it up, and serving.
- Bread making can be enjoyable as well as good hand therapy. Making rolls, bagels, coffee cakes, etc. is an interesting variation.
- A group having similar disabilities can share tasks and try out skills that might be difficult if done individually (e.g., one-handed persons trying to open boxes, jars, and cans, or mixing and stirring). Although the group coordinator should have some solutions ready, members may have techniques of their own to share, and the others may be more receptive to suggestions coming from a group member.
- Diet planning is helpful for those who need assistance or the support of a group in sticking to their diets. A dietitian can help with the planning and education, and the participants can fix the meal. A social worker can facilitate group understanding of the social and emotional needs that may interfere with members' compliance with their diets, can offer psychological support directly to the group, and can supply information about community supports for those on restricted diets.

KITCHEN FEATURES

If there is an opportunity to set up a kitchen:

- Make certain that there is adequate space for wheelchairs, including turn-around room.
- Provide continuous counter space between sinks and appliances to make sliding easier (important for those limited in strength and in capacity for lifting).
- Use stoves with controls located on the front to eliminate unnecessary reaching.
- Provide open counterspace for those who lack endurance in standing and who can utilize a high stool when they must sit down.
- Provide an open-skirted table where several people can sit comfortably. (A pedestal table works well.)
- Make certain that electrical outlets are located at counter level.
- Provide a refrigerator with a door that opens toward the counter space.
- Arrange basic equipment so that reaching is kept to a minimum.

A kitchen with low counters and cupboards is comfortable and efficient for the wheelchair user, but might prove awkward for ambulatory persons. Also, few persons can afford the luxury of this kind of modification in their homes. (Note: The disabled full-time homemaker may be eligible for financial assistance in home renovation from the local department of vocational rehabilitation, since homemaking is considered a vocation.

Chapter 10
Carry-over to the Home

The pathology of many disabilities may be irreversible, but the physical, emotional, social and vocational consequences need not be.
U.S. Senate Committee on Aging Hearings

Beyond the disabled person's need for abilities to carry on normal daily activities, there is the need for effective use of leisure time as well as for recreation and socialization. One of the main goals of a therapeutic activities program is to develop new interests and abilities with some carry-over to the home.

PRACTICAL USE OF ABILITIES

There is often an indirect benefit from developing abilities for daily living. The person who has relearned to prepare a snack, for example, can now invite a friend in for a visit and offer something to eat. New interests can expand and grow. For example, windowsill gardening can become a hobby and can provide a way for the gardener to make a gift of a terrarium or a new plant grown from a seed or slip. Painting is another such open-ended interest, as are handcrafts, and not all the new skills and interests are necessarily solitary activities or simply ways to pass the time. One activities program participant became so proficient at handcrafts that she now teaches what she learned to young mothers in her home. Another makes macramé hangers and sells them to supplement her income. Still others invite friends in to join in making various gifts.

For some participants, the activities program is an introduction to a new circle of friends. Many disabled people find it more comfortable to be with those who have also experienced a disability and who are geared to a slower pace.

FAMILY ASSISTANCE

The family is vital in aiding the carry-over of significant program activities to the home and in reestablishing as much independence as the disabled person can handle comfortably. As one program staff member put it, "The participant and the family need to work out a new contract on how they will all live together." Therefore, the more the family is involved with the program, the better for all concerned.

For instance, family members should learn how to help participants with the activities of daily living so as to facilitate their independence. It is particularly helpful for a family to become directly involved with new hobbies or projects, so that the disabled person is not left to carry out the activity alone. Above all, family members need assistance in understanding the limitations imposed by the participant's disability and the frustration that usually accompanies it. Disability always affects home life. In many instances, the effect is devastating. Some family members behave like heroes in the presence of the disability of another member. Others find themselves unable to deal with the added stress. A family that did not get along well together before the disability may now perceive the family situation differently and experience some improvement in relationships. On the other hand, the disability may bring with it so much threat that the relationships among family members are completely disrupted. In such instances, the disabled member who becomes involved in a therapeutic activities program could discover that such involvement has a healing effect, especially if some of the family members share in program activities.

When family members cannot facilitate the resocialization of disabled people and assist in meeting their recreational needs, the use of other resources is indicated. The number of community groups that welcome the disabled is growing. In one community, for instance, there is a club called the Able Disabled and another named the Handy Handicapped Stroke Club. Such groups may offer an opportunity for a continuation of what the person has learned in a therapeutic activities program while providing a socializing experience. The problem facing the potential participant is then one of transportation.

TRANSPORTATION

Door-to-door services using specially equipped vans are sometimes available commercially, but they are usually quite expensive. Most conventional transport services such as buses and taxis are not equipped for handling wheelchair users or even those who are less severely handicapped. Volunteers can help in some instances, as well as organizations such as the senior personnel employment agencies that are beginning to appear around the country. Transportation is sometimes available through community agencies.

THE COMMUNITY

Despite the fact that many communities are reaching out in service to handicapped persons, many such persons are still isolated and homebound because of chronic illness or disability. Too many programs aimed at serving the disabled are in locations with architectural barriers that hinder or prevent the disabled from participating. Organizations serving the disabled and acting as advocates can increase community awareness of the need to remove such barriers. In some communities, volunteer groups are available for services in the home such as friendly visiting, simple crafts, etc. If they are given the necessary training, some volunteers find this a satisfying community service. Research indicates that no matter what the format or sponsorship, the stimulation and socialization of therapeutic activities programs can play a major role in preventing the deterioration that can come from the isolation and loneliness so many disabled persons face.

Part II

Chapter 11

Therapeutic Craft Activities

The activities described in the following sections have proved interesting and within the capabilities of most disabled adults. They need not be limited to any certain age group, and can be enjoyed by non-handicapped people as well. The description for each activity is preceded by a discussion of its therapeutic implications to guide the reader in selection of activities for people with various disabilities.

Each chapter also contains a list of the required materials. The last section in each chapter (*Adaptations*) suggests some special items to make the projects easier for those with more limited functions. The adaptations are intended to make the projects feasible for almost any member, and encourage participants to help one another. Such sharing can provide a stimulus for socialization, an important therapeutic element.

Most of the projects include ideas for variations. In some instances, the variations may be more suited to some people or groups than the primary model.

It is essential that the person who will be teaching the project make up a sample beforehand. This will reveal any potential difficulties and will enable the teacher to modify the procedure to make it more suitable for the participants. It will also indicate any parts of the project that need to be completed by the staff ahead of time. Furthermore, seeing the finished product is likely to create interest.

This sampling of activities represents only a small part of the possibilities. There are unending choices for the inventive person, and the advantage of these projects is their easy adaptability.

"Therapeutic" means "possessing healing power," and structuring is important in all these activities if the therapeutic goals are to be achieved. Appropriateness of activities to individual needs is also of prime importance. People vary considerably in their residual abilities, personalities, motivation, backgrounds, and adjustability, and the program should be planned accordingly.

Chapter 12

Projects for the Visually Impaired or Blind

Throughout this manual, suggestions have been made for adaptations of projects for the visually limited. For the person with the single problem of lack of vision, agencies responsible for training of the blind should be used for specific kinds of teaching. But the geriatric population is often limited in its use of these services because of other disabilities.

Some of the suggestions below appeared in an article by David Sevel and Mrs. J.A. Hart in the *American Journal of Occupational Therapy* XXIII, No. 4 (July-August, 1969) entitled "Occupational Therapy for the Hospitalized Eye Patient." These may assist those working with the multi-handicapped, visually limited individual.

WORKING WITH THE MULTI-HANDICAPPED

1. Help people to think of themselves as having a limitation that can be lived with, rather than as being dependent on others. Don't avoid the disability; talk about it; it helps in adjustment.
2. Remember that human contact is extremely important for the visually limited, to keep them in touch with the world around them. Orientation to hours, seasons, time, and place must be continuous. Share with the visually limited some of the pleasant things in life that they might otherwise miss by not being able to see.
3. Encourage participants to be as independent as possible in self-care and mobility. They may walk best using a wall for guidance. Different wall textures can give the visually limited points of reference for certain rooms doorways, etc. Ambulatory people may be able to profit from cane training. If such training is not feasible, a participant can hold onto the elbow of a sighted person. For those with a lower extremity disability, a walker is

usually better. An additional rail can be attached to the front of a walker to be used as a bumper.
4. Assist the visually limited in developing other senses to reduce frustration. Hearing is an important compensatory mechanism for the blind or visually limited. Help them to locate the source of sounds in a room. (A hearing test may be needed to evaluate the capacity to distinguish sounds.) Train participants to distinguish between thick and thin carpeting, grass, earth, and cement, and to feel the sun on the face, hands, and body. Orient participants to smells (the kitchen, the woodworking room, and sleeping rooms all have distinct odors). Orient them to a particular room by placing their hands on various objects to note the space relationships.
5. Use lights to help the partially sighted, for example, red, green, and yellow to distinguish different areas.
6. Include individuals in group activities around them, and encourage socialization with conversation, word games (e.g., Password), singing, etc.
7. Utilize activities that provide sensory feedback with textured materials, heavy yarns, large holes for lacing, braid-weaving frames, etc. Have participants handle different weights, shapes, etc., to assist in discrimination of the environment and to help them organize their thinking.
8. Before giving instructions for a project, orient the participants to the objects and tools and materials to be used, and store the items in the same place each time.
9. Give clear, consistent verbal instructions, such as for the starting position of the hands.
10. Use gross activities for the newly blinded to help them develop their sensitivity of touch. It is especially important to use gross-textured materials for those who have poor touch so they can understand what the completed project is like. (Samples of items are very important.)
11. Use guiding devices such as:

- measuring tape stapled at intervals
- textured markers, such as raised-line rulers or yardsticks available from the American Foundation for the Blind (see Appendix E)
- tongue blades, notches, or tapes to define the limits of the working space
- different thicknesses of pegs, smooth and round surfaces, large pins, deep cuts on boards, and raised lines, spots, and surfaces (note Hi-Marks, Appendix E, for creating raised surfaces)
- clothing markers with different textures to indicate the nature and color of garments, or Braille markers, available from The American Foundation for the Blind (see Appendix E).

Projects for the Visually Impaired or Blind

12. Use craft activities in which the participants can feel the completed project. Painting, block printing, or silk screening would be poor choices because the results cannot be felt.

    Initial Activities: braiding, finger weaving (using a single color or different textures for different colors), mosaics, Turkish knotting, one-piece wood projects (cheese boards, vegetable cutting boards, or racks for coat hangers), copper-tooling molds, pine cone projects, etc.

    Later Activities:

    - knitting (use short needles, a stapled tape measure, and cardboard cut in the shape to be knitted)
    - ceramics (glazing is difficult; use one color and have the participant mark the starting point, then work from the top to the bottom and repeat several times)
    - loom weaving (teach the participant to feel spaces and edges, pin a tape measure to the starting point, and mark with a pin where the work should end)
    - loopers—with the woven part towards the participant
    - link belts (point out the contrasting textures of front and back)
    - leather-lacing projects—with large holes and rubber cement to hold the pieces together (short lacings are best, since they are less likely to twist, and contrasting colors are best for the partially sighted).

13. Use writing aids, such as a piece of heavy cardboard with lines punched by an awl or a sewing machine, or rubber bands run across horizontally, stabilized on notched edges. The left hand stays at the beginning of the line; the right hand, holding a pencil, returns to the left hand and then drops down to the line below. "Right-Line" paper, also, can help those who need tactile clues. (See Appendix E.) For the visually limited, provide strong light and avoid projects that require close attention. For those with diminishing sight, select activities that do not require sharp vision. Participants can be encouraged to try gross activities blindfolded or with their eyes closed to improve their sense of touch.

THE ISOLATED PERSON

Blind people become isolated by choice or because of the lack of stimulation. Their wishes should be respected to the extent of allowing them to choose not to participate in group activities. However, if the lack of participation becomes detrimental to a person's psychological health (by causing depression, for example), a staff member should intervene with gentle persuasion. It is important to remember that the way an activity is presented may make the difference between participation and nonparticipation. For example, "We're going to be listening to music today. What's your favorite?" is better than "Would you like to go to the music group?"

BRAILLE, LARGE TYPE, AND RECORDINGS

Learning to read Braille is dependent on good memory and excellent sense of touch; its use is not appropriate for someone with diminished concentration, memory, or sensation. However, some geriatric persons can learn enough symbols to play some of the Braille games, such as cards or bingo, that are available from the American Foundation for the Blind. (See Appendix E.) Braille books are available through the Library for the Blind and Physically Handicapped. (See Appendix E.)

Such publications as the *New York Times,* the *Reader's Digest,* and other current magazines are available in large type to the legally blind through the Library Service for the Blind and Physically Handicapped. Most local public libraries stock large-print books, or will be happy to obtain them through interlibrary loan.

Talking Books and tape or record machines can be borrowed through the Library Service for the Blind and Physically Handicapped, Library of Congress, Washington, D.C. 20542. (See Appendix E.)

Chapter 13

Craft Projects

PAPER AND GLUE

Therapeutic Implications

The following activities have three requirements in common: cutting or tearing, gluing, and applying finish.

Decoupage, papier mâché and tissue-paper collage may be ranked as activities that require a minimum of coordination, while magazine page art requires fine dexterity and precision. They can all be classified as structured crafts, but contain an imaginative component in the selection of materials to be used. All of these can be used effectively as group projects. If some participants cannot cut with scissors, others can do it for them. Cutting is an excellent activity for those needing strengthening of the muscles that open and close the hand (finger extension and flexion). The weight of the scissors and the ease of opening them can be adjusted to meet the exercise requirements. If precision cutting is required, a paper cutter can be used for straight lines.

Decoupage

Since wood preparation is required initially, decoupage can be used to encourage gross muscle strengthening, and the distressing of a board can provide a healthy outlet for working off frustration. The repetitive nature of sanding and pounding is particularly appropriate for those who are limited in fine motor control or who have difficulty initiating motion. Lightweight hammers (a ball-peen hammer is good for distressing) can be used for those with limited strength, and tool handles can be built up with foam rubber to give a better grip. (See *Woodworking* for additional therapeutic implications.)

Since little vision is needed in this project, except for picture placement, it is a good one for a visually or perceptually limited person.

Papier Mâché

Papier mâché consists mainly of tearing or cutting strips of paper and placing them; this requires minimal muscle strength in at least one hand. The thickness of the paper being torn or cut can be varied to make the project adaptable for strengthening muscles. Tearing, as well as sanding or pounding, is good for the person who needs to vent feelings of aggression. Layering and overlapping of paper does not require good vision.

As papier mâché may have some association with elementary school days, the project should be carefully chosen, be useful, and be introduced with some degree of sophistication. Craft films and slides are helpful here, or an attractive completed project sample could be displayed.

Magazine Page Art

Magazine page art is beneficial for those needing a variety of small exercises for the muscles of the hand. It requires minimal to moderate muscle strength for grasping, releasing, and cutting. The rolling process calls for finger flexion and extension. Since a number of disabilities cause problems with finger extension (due either to joint limitations or to imbalance of muscle strength), rolling the dowel forward with the fingers straight is a good exercise to stimulate increased extension and to prevent flexor deformity.

The exacting nature of the gluing process and the necessity of rolling and accurate tube placement limit this activity to those with fair finger dexterity. It is excellent for people who have the potential to increase fine eye-hand movements. The tube placement is particularly good for the visually impaired, since the contrast between the can and the tube is gross and offers good sensory feedback.

For those needing more mental stimulation, the measuring involved in cutting the magazine pages is a good activity. A pattern can be used, of course, for those who are more impaired.

Spray finishes should not be used by those with respiratory problems.

Tissue Paper Collage

Tissue paper collage is physically less resistive to the grasping and holding required. Tissue is thin, and therefore requires greater dexterity in picking up the pieces than the magazine pieces that are used in other forms.

The overlapping method eliminates the need for precise placement. Tissue, however, allows little sensory feedback, so it is not particularly useful for the visually impaired; magazine pieces are preferable.

Decoupage

Materials

1. sandpaper
2. screwdriver
3. wood stains
4. latex paints, assorted colors
5. paintbrushes
6. scissors
7. brayer (roller)
8. waxed paper
9. paper towels or soft cloths
10. Mod Podge*
11. picture hangers
12. antiquing glaze (optional)
13. hammer, wood carving tools, nails, etc., for distressing wood
14. scraps of lumber
15. small boxes
16. bottles
17. trays
18. pictures cut from gift wrappings, greeting cards, magazines, family pictures, etc.

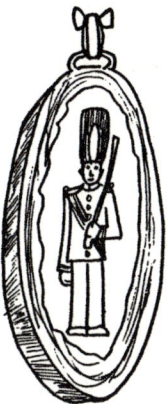

Figure 13-1

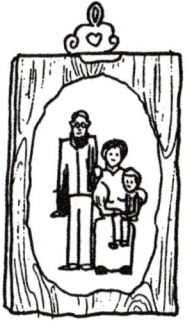

Figure 13-2

Procedure

Select the picture to be used, and a board on which to mount it. The board can be an oval (Figure 13-1) or a vertical (13-2) or horizontal (Figure 13-3) rectangle.

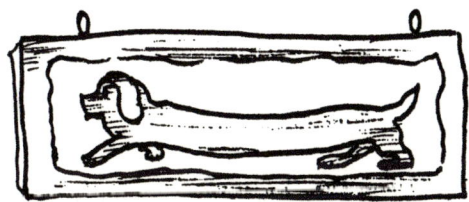

Figure 13-3

*Diluted white glue can also be used, but is less satisfactory.

Distress the board with wood carving tools and a hammer, making slashes, holes, hammer marks, and other damage to make it look old. Sand the board to remove the rough edges. Stain or paint the board to blend with the picture and put antiquing glaze on it when the paint or stain is dry. Wipe off the excess glaze with a soft cloth or paper towel. Allow it to dry thoroughly.

Cut out the picture, tear it around the edges, or cut it so that a margin of wood remains around the picture. Brush glue over the entire back of the picture, turn it over and center it on the prepared board, cover it with waxed paper, and use a brayer to remove air bubbles from under the picture. (Roll from the center out toward the edges.) If you cannot remove an air bubble by rubbing, prick it with a pin, allow the air to escape, then rub again.

When the glue is completely dry, coat the work with varnish. For a rich finish, apply several coats, allowing each to dry and sanding to remove all the bubbles. Apply the next coat, repeating the process each time. The picture will appear to sink into the wood. Use decorative hangers, available at most craft supply houses, to add an attractive finish to the completed project.

Cut-Work Variation

1. Prepare the wood surface as described.
2. Choose a print of flowers, fruit, or a figure.
3. Seal the entire print by coating it with a sealer of diluted white glue or a light coat of varnish. (Some latex varnishes can also be used as adhesives for paper and cloth.) Let the print dry.
4. With decoupage scissors (or nail scissors) carefully cut away all the background material from around the main design so that only the figure or grouping of fruits, etc., remains. Gently sand the outer edges of the print, from the back, so the print will "sink" into the wood and give the illusion of an original painting on wood.
5. Position and glue the print onto the prepared wood surface.
6. After the glue has thoroughly dried, apply several coats of varnish, sanding between each coat.

Adaptations

With the use of a C-clamp, a one-handed person can prepare the wood surface (distressing, sanding, and staining), but might need assistance in preparing the picture and applying it to the plaque.

Greeting cards or prints can often be used for pictures, as they require little or no cutting.

Boxes and other containers lend themselves well to the decoupage technique.

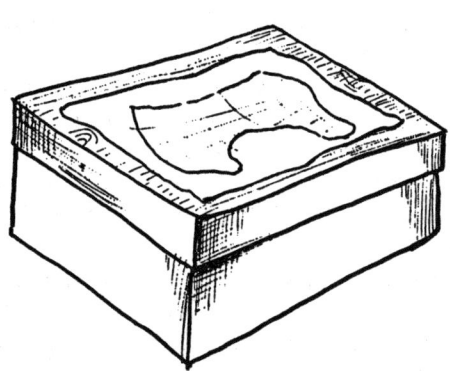 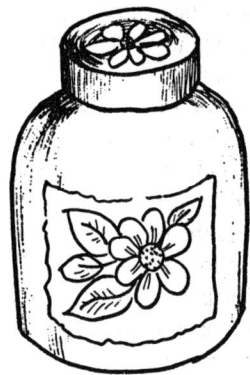

Working with Papier Mâché

Papier mâché, or paper mash, is one of the most versatile of art crafts. It is the art of creating decorative or useful objects with paper, from the simplest (such as covering a bottle or other container) to expressive sculpture. There are basically two techniques. One uses strips of paper, applied in layers, and the other uses paper mash the way clay is used.

Basic forms can be made of cardboard or throw-aways, such as coffee cans, containers of all sizes, or plastic bottles. Domed shapes (formed over balloons or lubricated bowls) can be used as molds.

The finished object can be decorated with paint, after coating and sealing it with gesso or diluted white glue, and the design and color possibilities are limitless. Felt, fabric, beads, edgings, etc., can be added for bright finishing touches.

The techniques for the two methods follow, with a sample project for each.

Papier Mâché—Strip-Dip Method

Strips are used

1. to cover a flat surface on trays, boxes, bottles, etc.,
2. to cover rolled or crunched paper that needs a surface for painting or decorating or to cover animals' bodies that have paper armatures,
3. to provide a surface for the application of gesso, glue, or mash so that painting or other decorating can be done, and
4. to act as tape in attaching ears, wings, tails, etc., to animals and figures.

Materials

1. wallpaper paste or white glue, for gluing
2. white glue or gesso, for sealing
3. bowl, or jar with screw-top, for mixing
4. water
5. newspapers, kraft paper*, and paper towels
6. brush for glue, 1″
7. paintbrushes
8. oil of cloves or oil of wintergreen
9. lacquer or quick-drying varnish

Procedure

Making Strips. Tear 1″ strips of newspaper, tearing with the grain (top to bottom for regular size newspapers, side to side for tabloid size). Do not use any cut edges of the paper (all paper used in papier mâché must have torn edges to make a smooth finish).

Mixing Glue. Wallpaper paste is mixed with water to make a glue of whipping cream consistency. Follow the directions on the package for proportions of powder to water. Use a jar with a screw-top and shake vigorously until a creamy mixture is formed. Add a drop or two of oil of cloves or oil of wintergreen as a preservative if the glue is not to be used up in one or two sessions.

White glue is diluted with a little water until it is of whipping cream consistency. (Oil of cloves is not required.)

Store glue in jars with tight covers between uses.

Applying Strips. There are two methods of applying the strips to the object to be covered:

1. The strips can be dipped in glue, one at a time, and applied to the object.
2. The strips can be dipped in water, one at a time, applied to the object, then brushed with glue.

In either case, after dipping, the strips must be run between the forefinger and second finger of one hand to remove the excess glue or water to prevent pooling of water around the object.

Apply the strips in layers in alternating directions to distinguish one layer from the other, to make the surface even, and to aid in counting the layers. Four layers are minimum; successive layers can be added for strength where called for. (A bowl or dish that will eventually hold objects of any weight should have six or nine

---

* Brown wrapping paper, grocery bags, etc.

layers applied.) Also, strips of kraft paper can be applied in layers once or twice during the process for added strength.

Check each layer to see that the paper is pressed down well and that creases and rough spots have been smoothed out to prevent the formation of air bubbles. This is a wet medium, so keep paper towels handy for soaking up any water that accumulates.

Finishing. When the surface is dry, seal it with a coat of gesso or diluted white glue. If twine is to be used for decorating, glue should be used as a sealer because gesso dries to a plaster-like finish and twine would slip on its surface. Gesso is good for a surface that will be painted, or where forms cut from cardboard, or other non-flexible shapes, are added for decoration. Apply three coats of lacquer or quick-drying varnish to the finished project for durability.

Papier Mâché—Mash Method

Mash is used

1. to cover flat surfaces for added strength,
2. to cover curved shapes (balloons, masks, etc.),
3. to add decorative shapes where needed,
4. to strengthen structures (by padding mash into corners),
5. to squeeze around narrow armature pieces where strips would give a clumsy effect, and
6. to work like clay in making small (3''-4'') figures.

Materials

1. newspapers (six double sheets, regular size)
2. glue (see *Strip-Dip Method* for preparation)
3. wooden dowel with 1'' or larger diameter, or wire whisk
4. vessel for soaking and boiling mash
5. water
6. sieve
7. trowel or spoon
8. lacquer or quick-drying varnish

Procedure

Making Mash. Tear the newspaper into 1'' strips. Tear these again into small pieces, place them in the vessel, cover with water, and let soak overnight. (If static electricity occurs in the tearing process, wipe the hands with a dry sheet of the anti-static paper product—Bounce, for example—that is used in laundry dryers.) Boil the soaked paper for twenty minutes to loosen the fibers. Pound the paper into a pulp with the dowel or beat it with a wire whisk. (If the full six sheets of newspaper are used, it will be easier to pound half of the quantity at a time, then combine for the rest of the process.) Strain and squeeze out most of the water, then stir in the glue mixture and mix together until the pulp can be squeezed into a shape and will hold a form. Store it in a tightly closed plastic bag until ready for use.

Applying Mash. Before applying mash to a surface, brush it with glue. Then trowel on the mash and smooth it with the trowel or the bowl of a spoon if large areas are to be covered. (It can be applied with the hand and pressed or squeezed into place when working on small pieces.)

The mash hardens to a very strong final stage and can be mended and added to after it has dried. Just remember to apply the glue before adding the mash for mending.

Finishing. When the surface is dry, seal it with a coat of gesso or diluted white glue before painting. Glue is preferred as a sealer if twine or fabric items are added as trim, because the gesso dries to a hard plaster-like finish and non-flexible material slips on its surface. Apply three coats of lacquer or quick-drying varnish to the finished project for durability.

Papier Mâché Bowl (Strip-Dip Method)

Materials

1. bowl-shaped container for a mold
2. glue (see *Strip-Dip Method* for preparation)
3. bowl for mixing
4. newspapers
5. kraft paper or paper bags
6. paper towels
7. lacquer or quick-drying varnish
8. acrylic paints
9. gesso
10. scissors
11. petroleum jelly
12. plastic wrap
13. brush for glue, 1"
14. paintbrushes
15. seine twine (will not shrink)
16. waxed paper to cover working surface

Figure 13-4

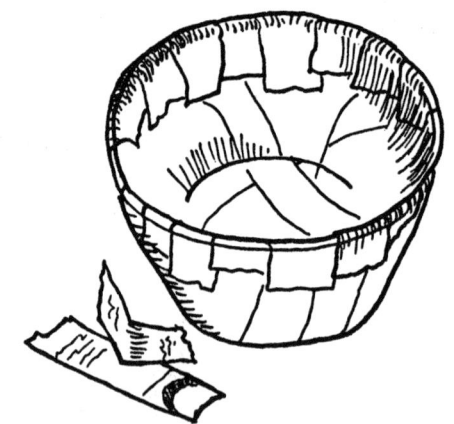

Procedure

Place the bowl to be used as a mold upside down on the waxed-paper surface. Cover the outside bottom of the bowl with petroleum jelly, then with plastic wrap, to prevent the glued strips from sticking to the bowl. (A layer of wet strips, without glue, will work as well as the plastic wrap.)

Begin adding newspaper strips dipped in glue (or dipped in water, then brushed with glue), covering the bottom of the bowl in one direction first. Alternate the direction for the second, third, and fourth layers. For the fifth layer, use strips of kraft paper to give added strength to the bowl, then add a final layer of newspaper or torn strips of paper toweling. There will be overlaps at the bowl edges, but these can be trimmed off later. Check each layer to see that the paper is pressed down well, and smooth out any creases to eliminate air bubbles (these cannot be corrected later).

When the form is dry, remove it from the bowl and trim the rim edges. A blunt knife might be needed to loosen the paper shape from the mold if it sticks.

The rim of the bowl now needs to be given a finished edge. Tear 1" strips of newsprint into 2½" or 3" lengths, dip them in the glue and lap them over the bowl rim, smoothing them on evenly and securely. Set the bowl aside to dry. (See Figure 13-4. Figure 13-5 shows the finished bowl.)

When the bowl is completely dry, brush on a sealer of diluted white glue. Let dry. Dip lengths of twine into the glue and add a decorative finish of swirls or petal shapes to the outside of the bowl, to the inside, or to both. When the twine is dry, apply a coat of gesso as a base for painting (or paint over the glue sealer), and paint as desired. When the paint is dry, apply three coats of lacquer or varnish for durability and to give the bowl a finished look.

Figure 13-5

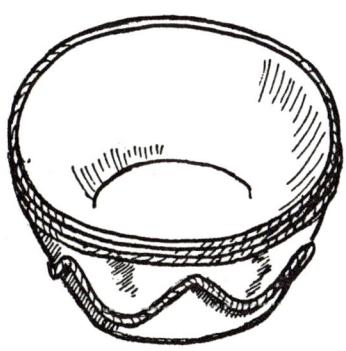

Decorating Variations

- Geometric shapes can be cut out of lightweight cardboard and glued on the bowl before the gesso is applied. This will give an embossed look to the bowl and will permit interesting options for painting (paint each shape a different color, etc.).

- Acrylic paint, from the tube, can be added to the gesso for a solid-color finish, then pictures can be applied after drying. Finish as usual, with two or three coats of lacquer or varnish.

- If a heavier bowl is desired, place the shaped bowl back on the mold, brush it with glue, and apply mash to cover it. A small pedestal base can be built up with the mash now, if the paper shape needs more support or more style.

Adaptations

- Use a flat plate or tray instead of a bowl for a mold.

- Anchor the mold to the table with tape or florist's clay, or put it on a Lazy Susan, for ease in handling.

- Use shorter sections of paper strips, dip them in the water, apply them to the mold, and brush with glue. Tearing paper strips will be possible for the one-handed if a brick is used to weight down the paper.

- For the mold, use a disposable plastic or paper item which can remain in the papier mâché.

Papier Mâché Swan (Mash Method)

Materials

1. mash (see *Mash Method*, p. 85, for preparation)
2. newspapers
3. pipe cleaners
4. twine or light-weight cord
5. white glue, diluted
6. gesso
7. white, yellow, and black acrylic paints
8. paintbrushes
9. lacquer or quick-drying varnish

Figure 13-6

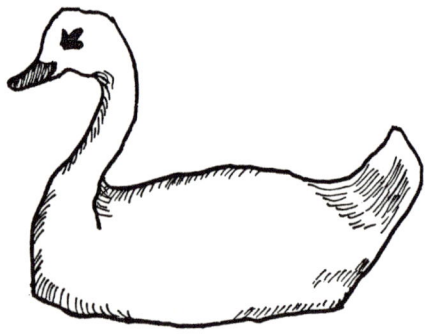

Procedure

Shape two pipe cleaners and dip them in glue. Let dry. (See Figure 13-7.)

When the pipe-cleaner armature is dry, crumple up some dry newspaper and fill in the body of the swan. Tie the newspaper in place with twine. Dampen the paper and pipe cleaners with glue and apply the mash to the swan's body, shaping by pressing the mash into place. If the neck of the swan causes problems, the body can be allowed to dry, then the mash can be squeezed onto the neck of the swan more easily. (See Figure 13-8 and 13-8a.)

When the swan is dry, apply a coat of gesso, then a coat of white acrylic paint if desired. Add the yellow beak and black eyes.

Figure 13-9 shows an armature for a four-legged animal. It was meant to be a horse, but turned into a camel during the mash application! (See Figure 13-10.) The same procedure as for the swan is used here: dip the shaped armature in glue, let it dry, then add the mash and squeeze it into shape on the armature. (A condiment can was used to support the animal's body while working with the mash.)

Figure 13-7

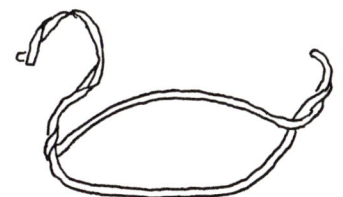

Figure 13-8

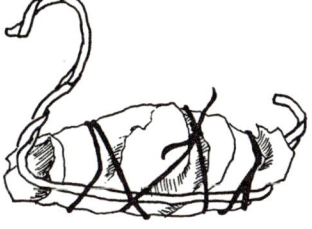

Figure 13-8a

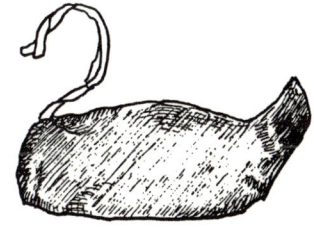

Figure 13-9   **Figure 13-10**

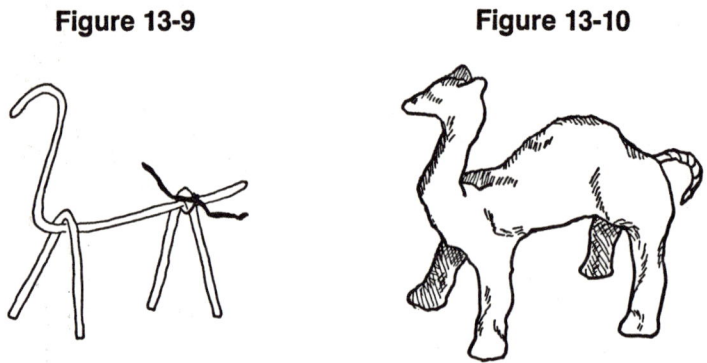

Beginners in handling this medium might want to make an animal in two stages: apply the mash to the legs, let it dry, then complete the body, neck, and face. The mash, when dry, becomes very hard; the legs will give good support for completion of the animal.

When the figure is dry, add whatever features are needed to complete it. Remember to apply glue to any surface that requires additions or mending.

Variations

Mash is a flexible medium that can be used to cover a surface by troweling on over wet paper, or used as clay for sculpturing. Impressions or designs can be pressed into the surface while it is wet.

Adaptations

An alternative project for participants limited to the use of one hand is the following: Choose a shallow dish with an attractive shape. Grease the inside of the dish with petroleum jelly, cover it with plastic wrap, and press the mash (about ¼" thick) into the dish with the bowl of a spoon, shaping it along the sides to the top of the dish. If moisture forms, blot it up with paper towels. Be sure the mash is compactly pressed. Allow to dry overnight. When the paper shape is dry, apply several layers of strips as in the strip-dip method; brush the mash with glue and apply the strips in alternating directions. Let it dry, remove it from the mold, trim the rim of the dish, and finish the edge as shown in Figure 13-5. Apply a sealer coat and finish by painting or other decoration.

Small pendants can be shaped with the mash. Make impressions in the mash with beads, then, when the pendant is dry, glue the beads in place after painting.

Tops of boxes can be decorated with mash. Any flat surface that can be suitably anchored will serve well as a project for a one-handed person.

Magazine Page Art

Materials

1. ¼" wooden dowel, 12" long, or a No. 10 knitting needle
2. white glue
3. scissors
4. brush for glue, 1"
5. paper cutter, if available
6. clear acrylic spray or clear varnish
7. old magazines (at least 23 colored pages)
8. juice can, any size

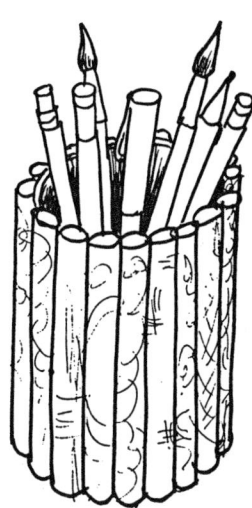

Procedure

Select colorful pages from magazines and trim off the white margins.

Measure the depth of the can, add 1", and cut squares this size from the magazine pages. (See Figure 13-11.)

For a 4" can, cut 23 squares, 5" on a side. (More, or larger, squares are required for larger cans.) Make a tube. Starting with one corner of a square, roll the paper around a dowel or knitting needle. (If a No. 10 needle makes too large a roll, use a No. 8.) Apply a small amount of glue to the last corner, and hold it in place until it is secure. (See Figures 13-12 and 13-13.)

Figure 13-11 Cut squares one inch larger than the height of the can.

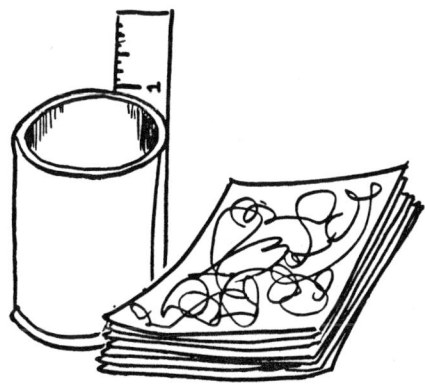

When the glue is dry, slide the rolled tube off the dowel. Continue making tubes until there are enough to cover the whole can. (They will be longer than you need and will be pointed at each end.) Now, cut about ½″ from one end. Place this end at the base of the can, just above the bottom rim. (See Figure 13-14.)

Now carefully cut the other (pointed) end so the tube will rest flush against the can and just beneath the upper rim. This tube is now a guide for cutting the remaining ones. When all the tubes have been trimmed, double-check the fit before gluing.

Figure 13-12 Roll the sheets around a dowel or knitting needle, starting at a corner.

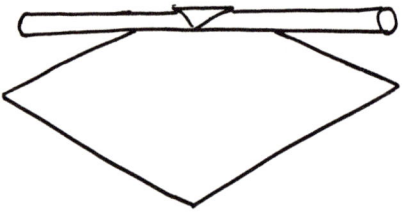

Figure 13-13 Place a small amount of glue on the last corner, and hold a moment until it is secure.

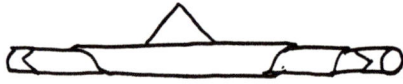

Figure 13-14 Fit tubes just above and abutting the bottom rim.

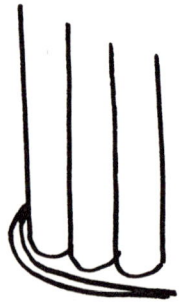

Most cans have a vertical seam. Put a line of white glue along this seam to use as a guide for getting the first tube exactly perpendicular. Place the first tube on this line of glue. Let it dry securely, and straight, on the seam. It will be worth the waiting time to have the first one straight and secure.

When the first tube is dry, apply a line of white glue alongside it and down the length of the can. (See Figure 13-15.) Put the next tube snugly against the first, and hold it in place until it is fairly firm. Repeat this operation all around the can.

Allow the work to dry thoroughly, then spray it with several coats of acrylic spray or brush on several coats of varnish.

Uses and Finishing Touches

- It can be used for a pencil holder or small flower arrangement.
- It can be turned over and used as a pedestal for a small plant or other object.
- Short pieces of plastic clothes line or sash-weight cord can be pushed into the holes at the top to form a scalloped edge. (See Figure 13-16.)
- The tops of the rolls can be crushed flat against the can for about ½" down, and an edging of cord or yarn wound around it.
- Experiment with other finishing touches.

Figure 13-15 First Tube at Seam

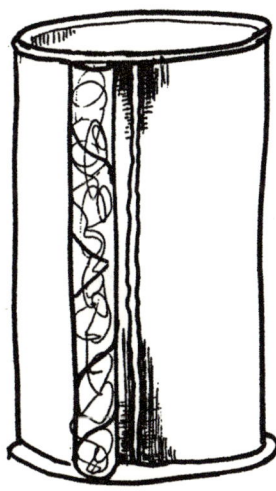

Figure 13-16 Scalloped Edge

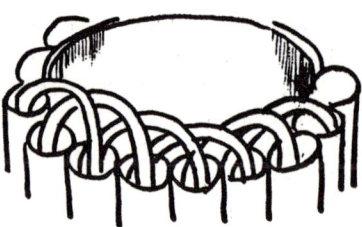

Variations

A five-gallon ice cream carton makes an attractive wastebasket. Paint or line the inside before gluing on the rolled paper.

Adaptations

The can could be anchored on its side with a C-clamp or cradled in a trough for gluing by a person with the use of only one hand. The pages can be cut by the one-handed if weighted down. (Consider using left-handed or electric scissors if cutting is difficult.) It is easier for a one-handed person to roll the tubes if the corner is properly lined up and the rolling is done slowly. For the visually handicapped, the first tube can be made by someone else to serve as a guide.

Tissue-Paper Collage—Vase or Lamp Base

Materials

1. tissue paper, assorted colors
2. bottles or jars with smooth surfaces
3. white glue
4. brush for glue, 1″
5. paintbrush for varnish
6. clear, quick-drying varnish or Mod Podge
7. scissors

Note: Metylan Art Paste (a powder to which water is added) may be used in place of white glue.

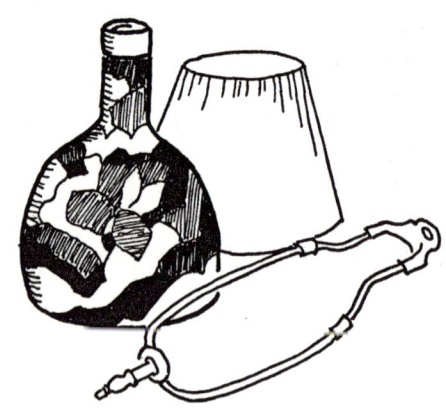

Procedure

Cut or tear tissue paper in various sizes and shapes. Apply glue to a small area of the bottle with a brush. Paste on a tissue-paper shape. Continue to apply glue and tissue paper shapes, overlapping previous pieces so no bare spaces show. Use random colors, or select colors that will give the desired effect when overlapped. Experimentation will develop patterns.

After the bottle or jar is covered, allow it to dry well before applying one or two coats of varnish or Mod Podge.

Lamp parts and a shade can be purchased to make an attractive lamp from a narrow-neck bottle. If the object is to be used as a vase, finish the rim with a band of tape or paint it.

Variations

- A raised or embossed effect can be achieved by crushing the tissue as it is applied.
- Pictures cut from magazines can be used in place of tissue paper. Themes can be developed by using pictures of public figures, sports figures, animals, flowers, etc.
- A stained-glass effect can be made by outlining the tissue-paper shapes with a heavy black felt marker after the glue is dry and before applying varnish or Mod Podge.

Adaptations

If a heavy bottle is used, the weight will be enough to hold it in place for a one-handed or weak person. A lighter bottle can be supported between slats of wood anchored to the table with C-clamps, or the bottle can be weighted with stones or sand.

The cutting can be done with the paper weighted, because the shapes do not have to be precise.

For the visually limited, a piece of masking tape or friction tape can be placed vertically on the bottle, as a guide for lining up the paper, or, if sensation is intact, the person can be taught to feel the difference in the spaces.

Final finishing can be done on a revolving stand, with a marker at the starting point, for ease in applying varnish.

PRINTING AND STATIONERY

Therapeutic Implications

Printing is a craft with broad appeal to both men and women. Techniques are varied, from the complex process of setting type and using a printing press to the use of stencils and silk screening and the more simple techniques of using hand-cut blocks.

The three crafts described here are included for their simplicity in use of materials and their potential for independent functioning for those limited in physical abilities. The crafts bibliography gives sources of information on silk screening, which is not included here (because of its complexity) but is worth noting as a good gross motor craft, particularly in the resistive motion provided in applying the ink across the cut stencil. Because of the precision required in cutting and applying stencils to the silk, this part of the craft is difficult for most people with disabilities affecting upper-extremity functions or vision. An added limitation in silk screening is the requirement for oil-base paints, which are preferable to use in the printing process but are not acceptable for some people with respiratory or skin problems.

Physically, the three crafts included here require good coordination and some prehensile and grasp strength. The cutting of Styrofoam or, particularly, vegetable blocks necessitates more strength and control than the marbleized art, which requires little pressure. As the blocks and vegetables, when cut, are turned over and pressed for printing, the more proximal motions of elbow and shoulder are used. The use of the brayer is particularly valuable for elbow motion, in both extension and flexion. Placing the block to the craft worker's side encourages side reaching as well as flexion and extension of the elbow. The observer should note that some people tend to use trunk motion, leaning toward the side, rather than using elbow or shoulder motion.

The vegetables or blocks can be cut by the staff or by participants with greater control, and the printing can be done by those who are more limited.

Minimal strength is required for marbleized note paper; since the crayons can be applied in random motions, fine coordination is not necessary. It is important, however, that the participant have enough control of hand and arm to avoid being burned.

For the more adept participant, the cutting required in finishing off the marbleized paper offers the more mentally stimulating process of measuring. Cardboard patterns can be used as a guide for those who are more limited, and a paper cutter can be used for straight cuts. The small size of the paper used makes cutting difficult for the one-handed person, although some can manage this if they stabilize one edge of the paper with a weight or tape while cutting. The gluing process can be done by most people. A corner or edge can be taped to make it easier for the one-handed person.

Anyone who is severely limited visually will probably find these crafts difficult, because there is very little opportunity to use the sense of touch.

As all of these crafts require some accuracy in placement, the ability to judge spatial relations is important. Guides such as rulers or wooden squares are helpful to some in positioning.

Psychologically, the repetitive motions of stamping blocks, rolling the brayer, or scrawling crayons meet the needs of the more limited person. These motions also suit those who have little patience for fine, precise activity.

For the person who can handle the cutting and designing of blocks, the more compulsive needs are met through the preparation of the printing blocks themselves.

The potential for group interaction is good with all these crafts, because they offer the advantage of socialization in sharing.

Printing with Styrofoam

Materials

1. Styrofoam blocks, Poly-Print blocks, or meat trays from the butcher
2. blunt tool for incising the design (nail, ball-point pen, or orange stick)
3. acrylic paint, assorted colors
4. brayer for spreading paint
5. tray for paint
6. paper, note cards, or drawing paper
7. scissors
8. newspaper to cover the work surface
9. rags for cleanup

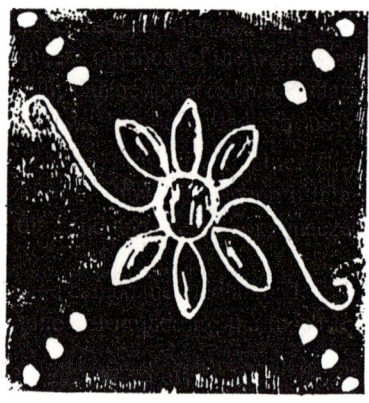

Procedure

With the blunt tool, press a design into the Styrofoam. (Meat trays from the butcher serve quite well if the commercial product is unavailable; they should be glued to a block of wood before using.) The raised parts between indentations form the design, which receives the paint and makes the impression on the paper.

When the design has been completed, pour the paint into the tray, run the brayer through the paint, then onto the surface of the block. Press the block on the paper, in the part chosen for the design.

Printing with Vegetables

Materials

1. raw potatoes, carrots, or other solid vegetables
2. paring knife
3. paper (various sizes) or note cards
4. stamp pads (assorted colors optional)
5. stamp-pad ink
6. waxed paper to cover work surface

Figure 13-17 Note Card

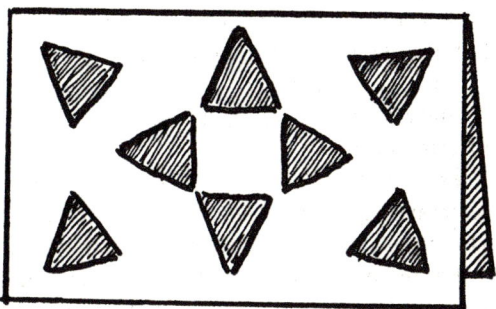

Procedure

Cut the vegetable to form a flat carving surface. Outline the shape on the flat surface. Incise the design by carefully cutting away portions of the vegetable around the design to leave a flat part raised for the impression to be inked. (Figures 13-17 and 13-18.)

Use the stamp pad to give an even coating of ink on the small surfaces of the vegetable design. (See Figure 13-19.)

An effective pattern can be made by repeated stampings of design, closely spaced, on a sheet of plain paper or a note card. (See Figure 13-20.) Gift-wrapping paper can be made by using large pieces of paper and repeating a design or combining one or more shapes scattered about. A single impression can be made for gift cards and place cards, or placed in the corner of writing paper to make it unique. A carrot is recommended for printing designs in small spaces.

Figure 13-18 Cutting Design

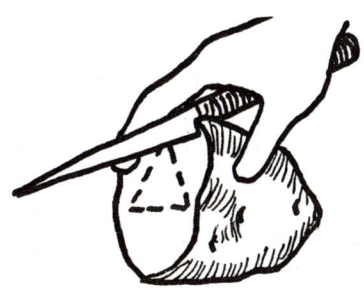

Figure 13-19 Ready to Print

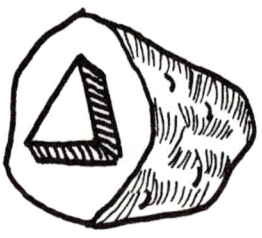

Figure 13-20 Printing

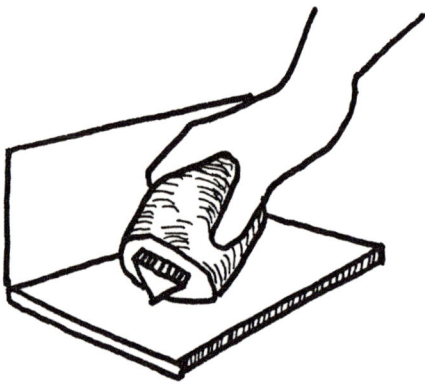

Variations

A standard fold-over note is 5½″ x 4¼.″ Use this measurement as a guide for note-paper designs.

Adaptations

The Styrofoam block can be taped to the working surface to stabilize it while incising the design.

Vegetables can be clamped in a small vise for carving and incising.

The Comfort Utensil Holder (see Appendix B) can be used to hold the tool for incising the design for those unable to hold the tool, or the tool can be built up with tape or foam.

If meat trays are used, it is advisable to run a clean brayer over the surface of the Styrofoam tray material before using it to assure a flatter surface for incising the design. The meat tray Styrofoam can be glued to a block of wood for easier handling.

Leaf Prints

Materials

1. freshly picked leaves with well-defined veins
2. paper, or polyester fabric
3. polymer medium, Liquitex
4. acrylic paints, diluted if too thick
5. paintbrushes, 1"
6. brayer or weights
7. waxed paper and newspapers for covering work surface

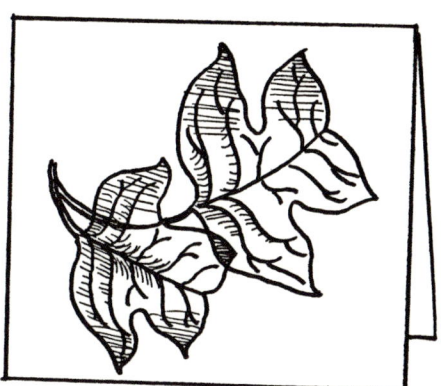

Procedure

Prepare the leaf surface by coating it with polymer medium.

Let the surface dry. Paint the leaf lightly with the desired color, then place it flat, with the painted surface down, on paper or fabric. Cover the leaf with waxed paper. Place a weight on it or use a brayer to apply pressure by rolling, being careful not to dislodge the leaf once it is placed in position.

After the paper or fabric has been imprinted, remove the waxed paper. Lift the leaf slowly, and allow the paint to dry before handling the print. The leaf can be washed and reused a few times before it has to be discarded. When the paint is dry, the paper or fabric can be finished by cutting (paper) or hemming (fabric).

After a few practice sessions, this printing process can be used to make a variety of items. A scarf, placemats, and other things can be made with polyester fabric (cotton cannot be used). Note paper, place cards, and gift wrap can be made with paper. See *Nature Materials* for information on card making.

Variations

Tempera paint and liquid starch mixed to the consistency of heavy cream can be used instead of acrylic paint, but the results will not be quite as satisfactory.

Adaptations

The leaf can be anchored to the working surface with tape for painting. Assistance may be needed with the paper cutting if note paper or cards are not precut.

Hemming can be done with the assistance of a one-handed embroidery frame attached to the table. (See Appendix B.)

Marbleized Note Paper

Materials

1. electric skillet (see *Variations*)
2. aluminum foil
3. scissors
4. ruler
5. paper cutter
6. rubber cement
7. old crayons, with papers peeled off
8. typing paper
9. note paper (about 4" x 5½") with matching envelopes
10. paper towels

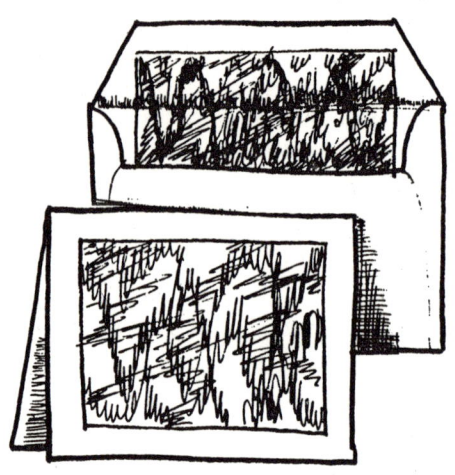

Procedure

Line the electric skillet smoothly with aluminum foil and heat it to 180° F. With the crayons, scribble different colors very heavily on the aluminum foil until an area as large as the typing paper is covered.

Make sure the skillet is hot enough to melt the crayons completely. Put a sheet of typing paper over the crayoned foil. With paper toweling in each hand (see Figure 13-21), blot the entire surface until a full coating of wax sticks to the white paper; then peel the paper off the foil and let it dry.

Figure 13-21 Blotting

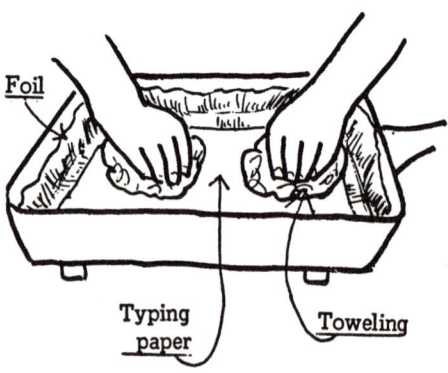

Look for interesting designs in the marbleized paper and cut it to fit the note paper. Leave a narrow margin around the edges, as you would for matting a picture. Glue it onto the face of the card with rubber cement. Then cut a similar lining for the envelope, letting some of it extend inside below the flap. Glue it in place with rubber cement.

Variations

This method can be applied to book marks, book covers, and gift-wrapping paper. As skill is acquired, more complicated projects can be attempted.

In place of an electric skillet, it is possible to use a hot tray, or a cookie sheet placed in an oven. If the wax cools, reinsert the sheet in the oven to blend the colors again.

Adaptations

A one-handed participant can apply the crayons to the foil, and do the blotting if the pan is warm enough to allow the crayon wax to flow freely without pressure.

Assistance with cutting may be needed.

A weight on the edge of the note paper and envelope will hold them in place for gluing, or this part of the project can be a team effort.

Caution

Heavy-duty extension cords must be used whenever an appliance cord is too short to reach a wall outlet.

BRAID WEAVING AND TURKISH KNOTTING

Therapeutic Implications

Weaving requires a fair amount of coordination in one hand and the ability to grasp a shuttle. If thread is to be carried by a needle or safety pin, finer grasping ability is needed. The size of the frame and its position (see *Adaptations*) determine the degree of shoulder and elbow motion used. A larger frame or one placed vertically instead of flat on the table encourages increased range of motion up to the shoulder. If the participant works from the bottom of the frame up, an increased reach is achieved. The warping, or winding of cord on the frame to begin the project, can be done with the frame in a horizontal or a vertical position; the vertical position necessitates greater shoulder range and the horizontal position requires more use of the elbow. As the weft yarn or thread is interlaced in and out of the warp thread, wrist action and elbow pronation and supination come into play.

Turkish knotting adds an additional challenge, as threads must be cut uniformly and placed for knotting in a consistent position. The threads can be cut one by one, utilizing resistive grasp and release of the hand, or by means of a thread block (see Figure 13-27). The block method can be done with X-acto knife, which requires less active grasp and release but more pressure in the proximal muscles. Turkish knotting can be done with one hand, although it requires good dexterity. It is a fine bilateral craft, considered to be moderately resistive. As the participant must pack the threads down or up, depending on which direction the weaving is going, finger extension and flexion are stressed alternately. A person who lacks power in the hand muscles tends to use shoulder and elbow motion to pack the threads. If the participant has active use of finger extension or flexion, stabilizing the elbow on the table while doing the packing will encourage better finger motion.

Weaving and Turkish knotting are structured and repetitive. Since they require the ability to alternate the shuttle (or needle or pin), sequencing is involved. The participant must be able to grasp the reversal process; this requires spatial planning and the ability to distinguish foreground from background. Directionality, as well as right-left discrimination, is involved. These crafts are good for training those who have visual field limitations, as it stimulates eye tracking and head turning (the frame and threads giving tactile cues). If different materials are used for the warp and weft, there is excellent tactile feedback.

These crafts are usually done individually, so there is little possibility for socialization. The projects are usually long-term, therefore not good for someone who needs more immediate satisfaction. They require concentration, and are a poor choice for the person who needs constant cueing because of poor memory.

Weaving

Weaving is basically the running of something in and out through some material. Projects such as baskets, looper potholders, and huck toweling embroidery all incorporate weaving techniques, as does weaving done on various types of frames.

Loom weaving can be done on a straight frame, in which yarn, cord, or thread is interlaced across vertical threads by hand, or it can be done on a table or floor loom, in which threads are lifted by pressing a bar or lever to create interesting patterns. The table and floor looms offer many therapeutic advantages because of possible adaptations for more resistance to shoulder, elbow, and (in the case of floor looms) lower extremity exercise. The disadvantage in their use is that more equipment is required and the warping (measuring, arranging, and threading) is very time-consuming and usually must be done by a staff member.

Braid weaving as discussed here can be done with less equipment, is easily adaptable to various set-ups, and has the potential for independent work by the participant.

Turkish knotting can be used in combination with braid weaving to add complexity and make the project more interesting.

Braid Weaving

Figure 13-22

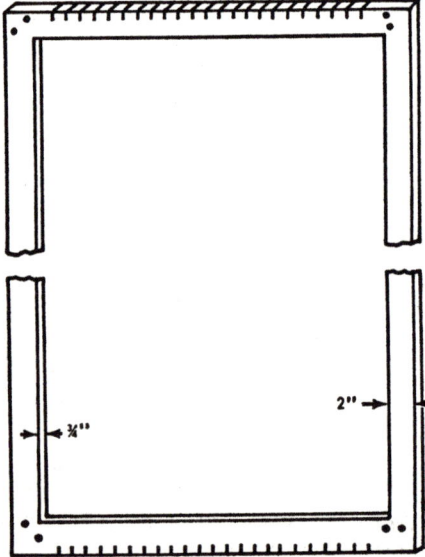

Materials

1. Braid weaving frame, purchased or constructed as in Figure 13-22. Width and length of frame are variable. Nails may be used at top and bottom instead of slots, but are more dangerous. Slots or nails are ½" apart. Frame should be glued and screwed together.
2. Scissors.
3. Flat shuttle, large safety pin, or large-eyed needle.
4. Heavy string or warping thread. Cotton or acrylic yarns are best for fillers, as shrinkage is minimum.

Procedure

Warping a Braid Weaving Frame. (See Figure 13-23.)*

Threading the Frame. (See Figure 13-24.) Step 1: The normal procedure is to fill the first two inches with cardboard, weaving in and out to give a base or heading to pack the yarn against. Step 2: Next, six rows of fine weaving material should be woven in to make the rug firmer and have a base for fringe (if preferred). Step 3: The yarn is passed horizontally on a wooden shuttle, or with a large safety pin or large-eyed, blunt needle. Step 4: The yarn is run over and under, then the order is reversed coming back. To start the end is split, so that one half stays in back and the other runs to the edge, looped under one thread and back under and over the same threads until it meets the other split thread. (All beginning threads should be in back.) If each new thread is started this way, the ends can be cut off without any danger of the piece disintegrating. Step 5: New colors or different weight threads may be added to give interesting design effects. A design may be planned in advance and, if complicated, tacked or taped to the top of the frame, hanging loosely behind the warp (vertical) threads. The weft threads may also be braided as they are run through (contrasting colors of yarn twisted between every warp thread), one color going over, one under.

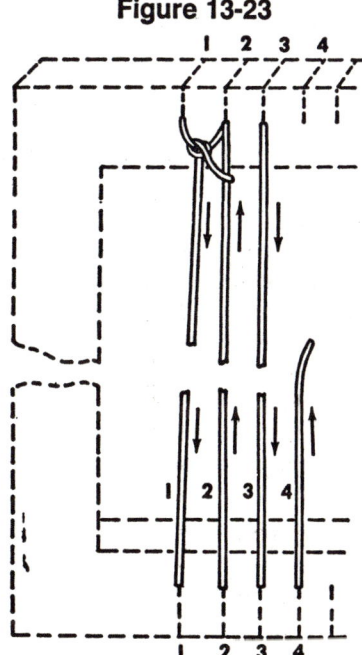

Figure 13-23

*Figures 13-22 through 13-29 are from TM8-290, *Craft Techniques in Occupational Therapy*, by permission of the Office of the Surgeon General, Department of the Army.

Figure 13-24 Threading the frame.

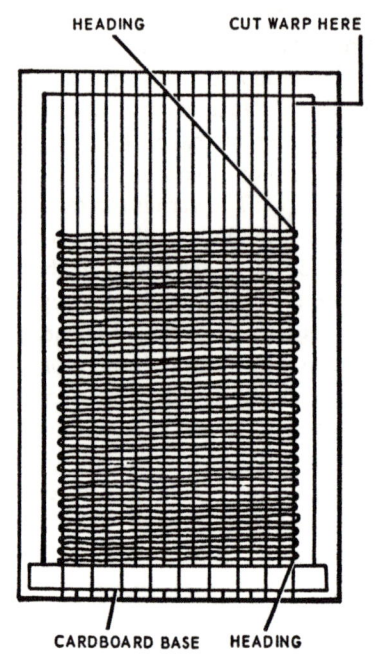

Top and Side Views. (See Figure 13-25, A and B.)

Method of Braid Weaving. (See Figure 13-26.) Rug-Stay can be sprayed on the back of the finished piece to prevent yarns from loosening, or a coat of diluted white glue (half water, half glue) can be brushed on the back. (These methods are usable only for something that will not be washed frequently.)

Figure 13-25

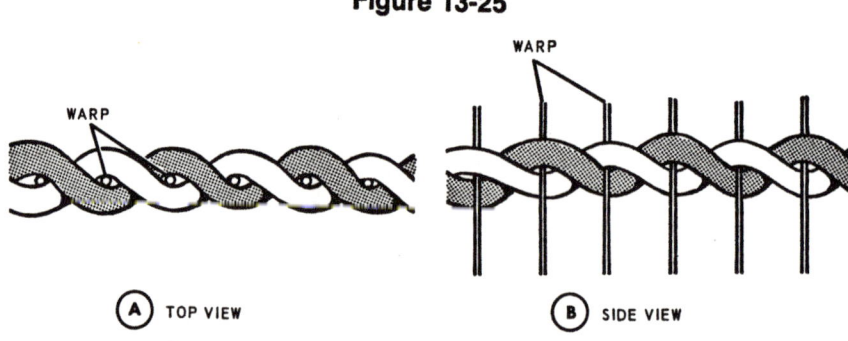

Figure 13-26

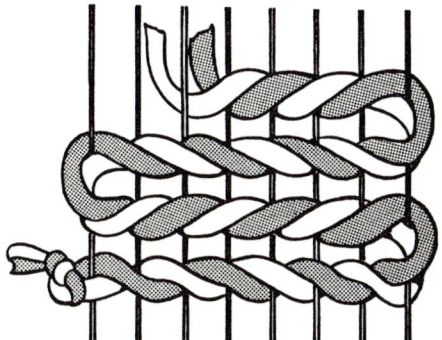

Turkish Knotting

Materials

1. The same weaving frame may be used for Turkish knotting, and adds more possibilities for exercise and design.
2. Material for Turkish knots should be heavier than tabby (the material used for over-and-under in weaving), and cut in 3″ to 5″ lengths, depending on how heavy the completed work is to be.

Procedure

Cutting the Lengths. (See Figure 13-27.) The lengths for the knots can be cut in one of two ways, wither by winding the thread on a piece of wood and cutting with a knife or scissors down the slot (as illustrated) or by marking the desired length on the frame and having the participant cut the lengths separately. The advantage in the latter is the grasp and release motions (if desired).

Figure 13-27

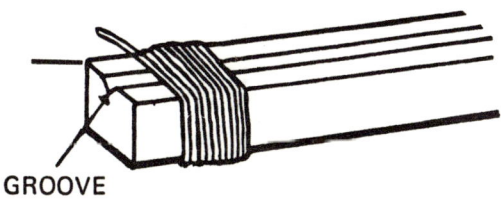

GROOVE

Tying a Turkish Knot. (See Figure 13-28.)

Plan of Rug. (See Figure 13-29.) The knots are run across one row; on the next row, the opposite threads are knotted so that spaces are filled in. After two rows of Turkish knots, two rows of tabby (over-under yarn), of lighter material, are put in.

Figure 13-28

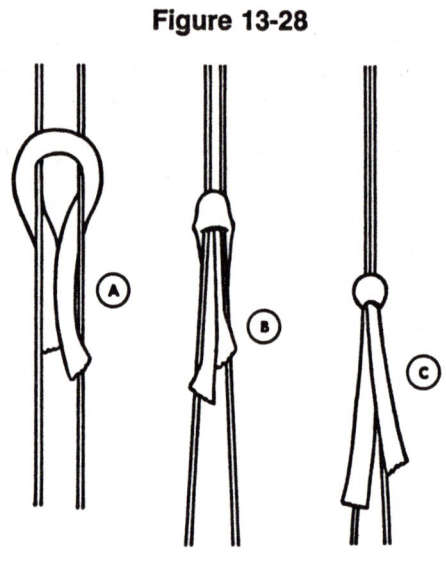

Figure 13-29

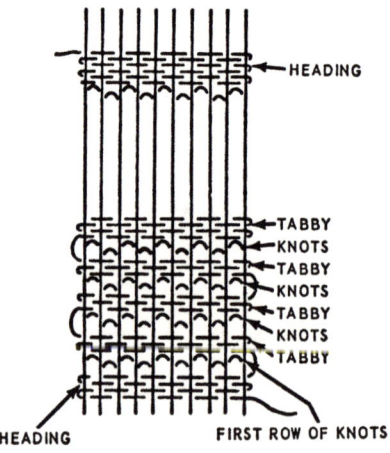

Adaptations

- The vertical (warp) threads can alternate in color or weight to make it easier for the visually impaired.
- Frames can be made in various sizes. Since knotting of large pieces is a long-term project, a small frame for an eyeglasses case, a small pillow, etc., may have more appeal for some participants.
- The frames may be adjusted in height with wood vises, easels, elevated boards, etc. To encourage reaching, longer shuttles can be used, but are difficult for the visually impaired or confused person.
- One color is best for the visually impaired or easily confused participant unless the shuttle or needle can be notched or taped. For someone with a good sense of touch, varying weights of yarn can be used for better orientation and an interesting texture.
- Special scissors may be needed for a participant working with the left hand. (See Appendix B.)
- Carrying the yarn on the shuttle will make for less cutting and eliminate needle threading. The shuttle can be clamped in a wood vise for one-hand wrapping.

STRING ART*

Therapeutic Implications

This craft is valuable for both the physically and the mentally impaired. It is easily adapted and requires little expense for tools and materials.

The physical requirements are as follows:

1. Muscle exercises for strengthening and range of motion are provided to the shoulder and elbow through the resistive activities of preparing the board, which may include sawing, sanding, and finishing (see *Woodworking* section for more details), or tacking or stapling the fabric to the board. Hammering nails utilizes wrist and shoulder motions.
2. Gross strength is required in one hand to do the sanding and make holes for pre-starting nails.
3. Fine dexterity is required in placing nails or pins at exact intervals. This is not appropriate for the person with more than minor coordination problems.
4. If wire is used instead of string, added strength is required for grasping and holding.
5. A graded range of motion (resistive against gravity) is possible for the shoulder and elbow: the higher the work is placed for stringing, the more shoulder motion is required. Placing the work on an inclined board also stimulates shoulder motion. If the work is positioned to one side, the elbow range can be increased. (For a right-hander, placement to the right encourages more elbow extension; placement to the left necessitates more elbow flexion.)
6. Perceptual skills are encouraged through tracing and placement of the pattern, and the stringing, involving:

   - directionality—the string is wound in a pattern, up and down, back and forth, clockwise and counterclockwise
   - depth perception—judging height and placement of the nails
   - figure-ground sense—discriminating between different colored strings and nails and the background

---

*The string art designs in this book were created by staff members of Burke Rehabilitation Center.

- spatial relationship—judging spacing of nails and string
- eye-hand coordination—locating numbered nails and following written or visual design directions.

7. Visual field limitations require compensation by turning one's head; training for this is encouraged through this craft, particularly where large patterns are used and the string goes from one side to the other. (If the participant is unaware of the field deficit, the work should be placed in the good visual field at the beginning.) A useful trial activity, to precede string art, is doing a follow-the-dot design. The difficulty of the string art can be judged by performance on this task.

8. Visually limited persons may be frustrated by this activity unless they have fine touch discrimination and good spatial awareness. A simple project, such as the practice circle (following) can be tried. Nails can be taped or painted on top to make it easier to locate them.

9. One-handed people can do this work independently if they do not have serious perceptual or visual problems.

10. Impaired language ability affecting reading or comprehension of numbers can cause problems in reading instructions and discriminating appropriate numbers. Pattern-tracing paper can be color-coded (the first layer marked with blue lines, the second layer with red) and a visual demonstration given. Simple repetitive patterns are best, such as No. 1 to No. 3 to No. 1 to No. 5, to No. 1, etc.

Mental Requirements

String art requires the ability to follow and retain written or verbal directions. It requires concentration. Because there are several different processes involved, it stimulates learning.

Psychological Factors

Because string art calls for attention to detail, it is not suitable for the easily distracted person or the one who cannot remember directions. It can be a relatively short activity, giving satisfactory results fairly soon, but a person who tends to be impulsive is likely to become easily frustrated because the strings can pop off the nails or pins if the winding is not done slowly and deliberately.

Practice Circle

Materials

1. pine or plywood, 12″ × 12″, at least ½″ thick
2. nails, flat-head, 1½″ or 2″ long
3. hammer
4. sandpaper
5. shellac
6. paintbrush
7. yarn or twine
8. marking pen

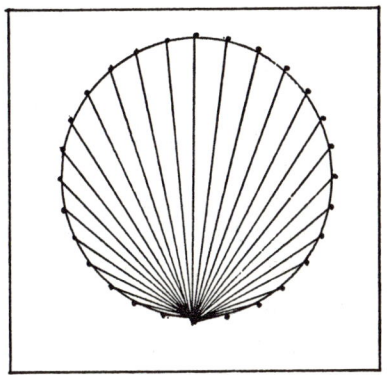

Procedure

Sand and shellac the board. Draw a 10″ diameter circle on the board and mark off spaces around the circle at intervals of about 1″ for an even number of nails (about 28). Hammer the nails securely in place around the circle, and number them, starting at the bottom center with No. 1. (See Figure 13-30.) Continue clockwise with No. 2, No. 3, etc. Also, indicate in some manner the top and bottom of the board. (Since the board is meant for re-use, a staff member should be responsible for setting up the board.) The measurements given here are only suggestions.

With the yarn or twine, tie a knot on the No. 1 nail and set up the order for the participant to follow around the circle (1-2, 1-3, 1-4, etc.), always wrapping the yarn around the nails in a clockwise direction and returning to the inside of the No. 1 nail before proceeding to the next number in the sequence. (If wrapping counterclockwise, return to the outside of the No. 1 nail before proceeding. It is important to be consistent; do not combine clockwise and counterclockwise wrappings in the same project unless the directions call for it.

When the yarn is returned to the No. 1 nail for the final wrap, a loose knot should be tied and the work should be checked for proper stringing. The yarn can be unwound and the same sequence of wrapping tried once again. Another selection of numbers can be chosen: 6-7, 6-8, 6-9, around the circle. Or, start at No. 1 and wrap just the odd numbers; then wrap the even numbers (1-2, 1-4, 1-6, etc.) with a different color yarn for contrast. This will give a two-level look to the work.

116 Therapeutic Activities for the Handicapped Elderly

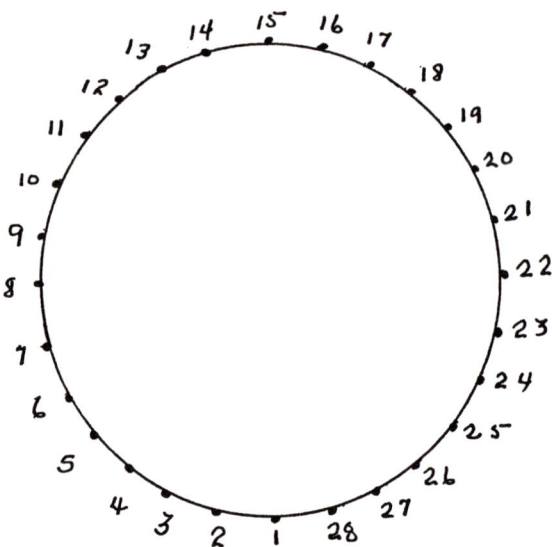

Figure 13-30 Nail Pattern

More elaborate numbering formulas can be set up once the simple steps of wrapping and following a numbering sequence are understood.

The participant who prefers a permanent piece of work can use a pattern for the design and work it on a covered or painted board (as described for the triangle string project, following).

Adaptations

- Use a C-clamp to anchor the board to the working table.
- Put the string or yarn in a large bowl or can to keep it from rolling off the table.
- Note that the precision wrapping described here does not have to be followed by those using the board for coordination exercises.
- Use layers of wrappings, in contrasting colors, for participants needing more challenge than one-layer work.
- Tape a tissue circle inside the nail periphery with directional lines marked from left to right for the more seriously impaired.

Equilateral Triangle

Materials

1. 10" square board (pine, flakeboard, or plywood, more than ¼" thick)
2. brads or linoleum tacks, ⅝" to 1"
3. hammer
4. paper for pattern
5. pencil
6. scissors
7. X-acto knife
8. tweezers
9. white glue or clear nail polish
10. paint, stain, or fabric (felt) to cover surface of board
11. string (crochet cotton) in three colors
12. hardware and wire for hanging

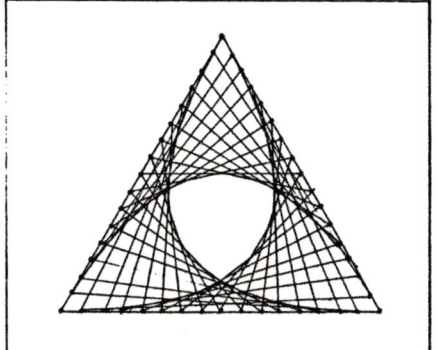

Procedure

Prepare the board by painting, staining, or covering it with fabric.

Draw an 8" equilateral triangle on paper, mark dots along the lines at ½" or ¼" intervals, and number these points as shown in Figure 13-31.

If desired, use tracing paper and copy the 8" triangle pattern, with points at ½" intervals. (See Figure 13-31.)

Center the triangle pattern on the board and tape it in place. Hammer brads securely in each point on the pattern, then carefully cut along the broken lines (as shown in Figure 13-31) with an X-acto knife and remove the excess paper. This will simplify the removal of the pattern from the board after the wrapping is completed. (The excess paper could be removed before nailing the pattern in place.)

Figure 13-31 Nail Pattern

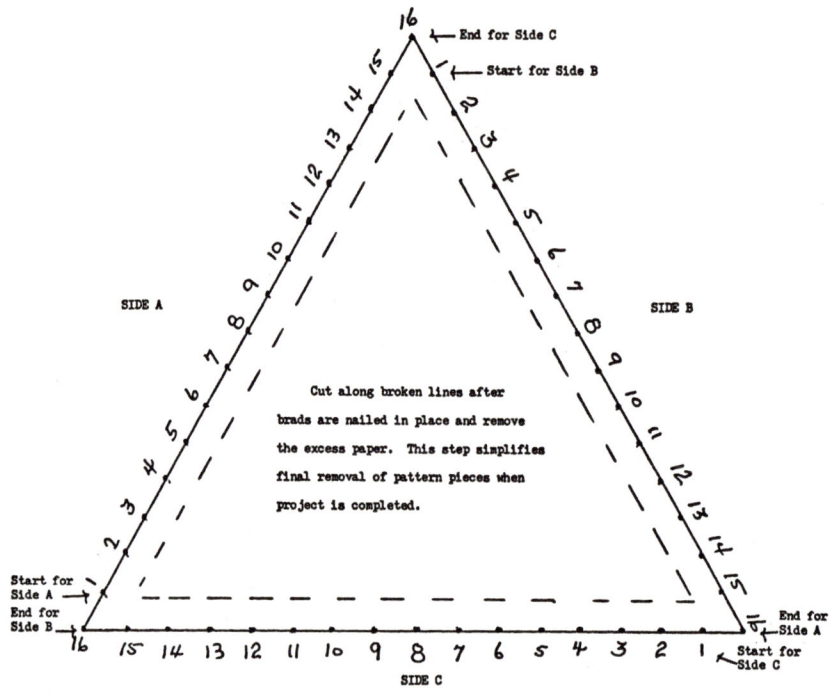

Stringing the Triangle. (See Figure 13-32.) With color A (A should be light, B medium, and C dark), tie the string on the No. 1 brad on side A of the triangle (leaving a 3″ length of string for final finishing) and wrap the string counterclockwise around brad No. 1 on side B. Return to No. 2 on side A, always wrapping counterclockwise around the brads. Continue in this manner until reaching "End for side A." Tie the string, leaving a 3″ length for final finishing.

Repeat this procedure for side B, using color B, and for side C, using color C. When the stringing is completed, put glue or clear nail polish on all the knots. Allow to dry before cutting the string ends. With an X-acto knife and tweezers, carefully remove the pattern paper from the board.

Variations

- Use metallic thread or yellow monofilament fishline on a black or red felt background, on a larger board with a larger triangle.

Craft Projects 119

Figure 13-32

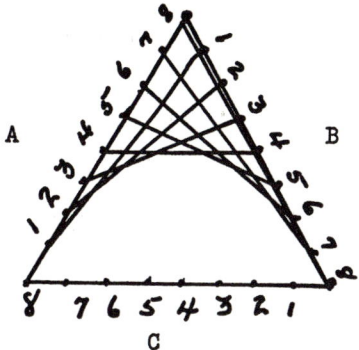

1. String side A-1 to side B-1

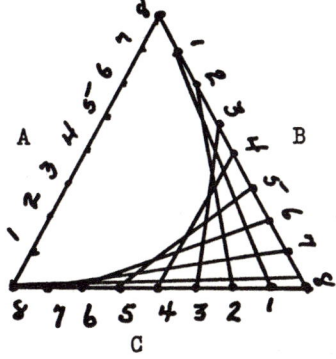

2. String side B-1 to side C-1

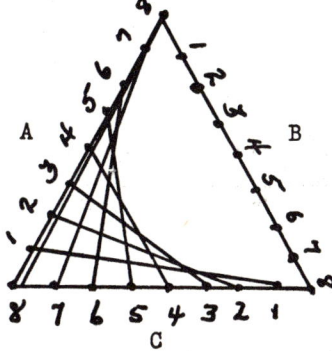

3. String side C-1 to side A-1

- Combine the practice circle, the triangle, and sections of the triangle in smaller sizes scattered on a contrasting background.
- Use different weights of stringing material for each of the three sections in the triangle.
- Experiment by drawing lines and curves, putting in points, and connecting them with pencil lines until you get an attractive free-form design. A ruler, compass, and protractor are helpful in line drawing and point placement. Color, texture of stringing material, background choice, and size are made-to-order ingredients for experimentation.

Adaptations

- The adaptations given in the *Woodworking* section can be used for making the board.
- Nails can be long (1½" or more), with flat heads, and spaced at greater intervals.
- If the stringing is interrupted, the string can be wrapped around one of the nails several times, and loosely tied, to keep the work from slipping.

Craft Projects 121

YARN WINDING

Therapeutic Implications

Yarn winding is light, repetitive, and structured. This makes it excellent for the person with generalized weakness or poor endurance. It requires light grasping and light prehensile ability in at least one hand. For the greeting card holder (following), use of the second hand in receiving the yarn passed through the can encourages assistive grasp. Some elbow action is necessary, and the range varies, depending on the size of the can and the work placement. Those with mild coordination difficulties can usually handle this, because they can stabilize an elbow on the table for greater control. Little shoulder range or strength is necessary, although shoulder reaching can be encouraged if the can is clamped in a vise. The contrast between the can and the yarn gives the visually limited a good tactile sense for foreground-background discrimination.

Some participants who have difficulty initiating motion can do the wrapping if an instructor first gives them hands-on guidance in the repetitive motion. Those with limited concentration and poor memory usually can do this craft, as it involves few steps.

Greeting Card Holder

Materials

1. juice can, large (No. 10)
2. yarn, four-ply nylon or acrylic (for Christmas, use red or green)
3. scissors
4. can opener
5. cardboard
6. yarn needle
7. construction paper, contact paper, or paint
8. white glue
9. small piece of popsicle stick or dowel
10. artificial holly and berries or artificial flowers and ribbon

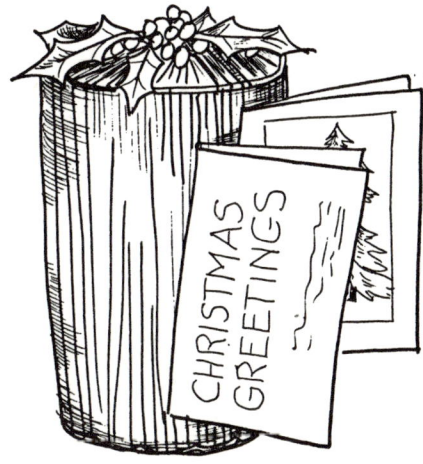

Procedure

Remove the bottom from the empty juice can and put the bottom disc aside for use later. (See Figure 13-33.)

In order to avoid having a shiny surface show through the yarn, cover the outside of the can with construction paper, contact paper, or paint. (See Figure 13-34.)

To start covering the can, roll the yarn into a ball that will fit into the opening of the can. Push the ball through, holding the end. Bring the ball around over the outside and tie the yarn with a knot inside the can. (See Figure 13-35.)

Figure 13-33 Can with Top and Bottom Removed

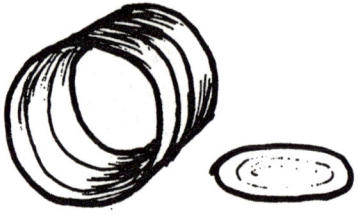

Figure 13-34 Covering Can

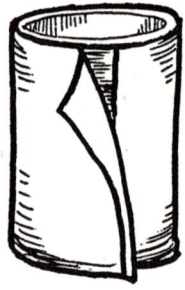

Figure 13-35 Tying the Yarn

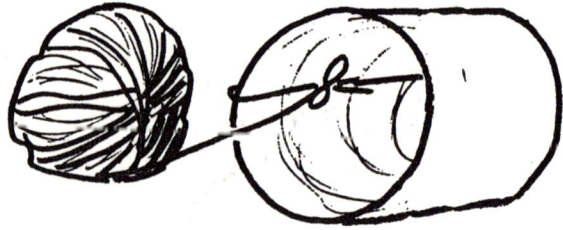

Continue pushing the yarn ball through and around, keeping the yarn strands close and taut. (See Figure 13-36.)

When the can is completely covered, tie a knot on the inside and cut the yarn.

Making the Cover. (See Figure 13-37.) Use the cut-out bottom of the can as a pattern for a circle traced on a piece of cardboard. Cut out the circle. In the center of the disc, make another circle about the size of a quarter, and cut this away from the larger circle. Cover both sides of the cardboard circle with the yarn, using the same over-and-under process as for the cylinder. Use long pieces of yarn instead of a rolled ball.

Figure 13-36 Wrapping the Yarn

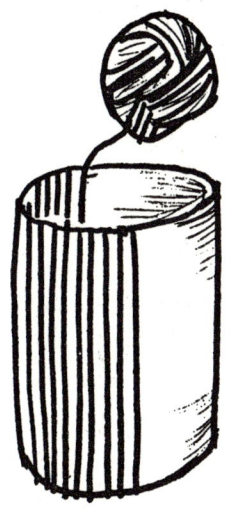

Figure 13-37 Making the Cover

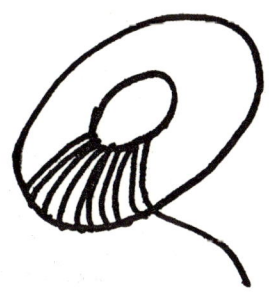

When the circle is completely covered, cut off the yarn and knot it on what will be the wrong side.

Finishing. (See Figure 13-38.) For a Christmas card holder, gather sprigs of holly together and push the stems through the hole in the center of the disc. Attach the protruding stems to the dowel or popsicle stick with wire or cord and place the lid on top of the finished juice can.

To attach the cover to the can, thread a yarn needle with the same yarn and stitch the cover to the top edge of the cylinder, taking alternating stitches about half an inch apart in the cover and at the rim of the can. (See Figure 13-39.)

For the year-round card holder, artificial flowers, fruit, or ribbon bows can be used instead of the Christmas decoration. As cards are received, they are opened at the fold and placed under a strand of yarn so the face of the card is on view. The holder is attractive, and displays many cards in a minimum of space.

Figure 13-38 Holly Decoration

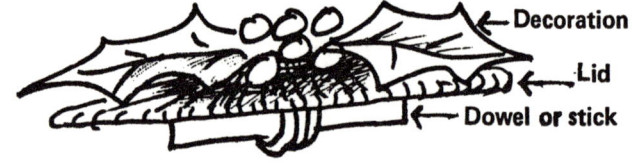

Figure 13-39 Stitching Top

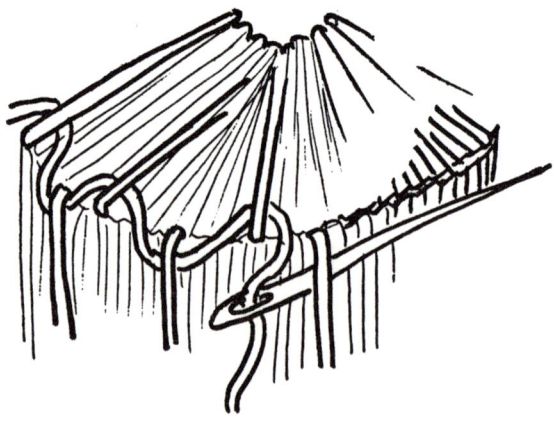

Variation

For a candy container, follow the preceding directions but do not attach the lid to the cylinder. Cut two cardboard circles. Finish the second circle without decoration and with a center cut-out smaller than the quarter used for the top and just large enough to permit the winding process. This is the bottom, and should be stitched on as described for the Christmas top. The container will have a decorative lid and a stitched-on bottom, and can be used for holding any light items (paper-wrapped candy, etc.).

Adaptations

Place the can on its side and anchor it to the table with a C-clamp. The clamp is moved as the work progresses. (Some assistance with tying knots and with the finishing steps will probably be needed.)

STITCHERY

Therapeutic Implications

Stitchery is a term applicable to many different crafts utilizing thread and needles; it includes knitting, crocheting, embroidery and needlepoint.

As crocheting and knitting require for the most part good dexterity, fairly good vision, and the use of two hands, they are not included in this text. However, they should not necessarily be eliminated from an activity program. Three factors should be considered when suggesting them to a participant:

1. They are both static activities that require little motion of the muscles that open and close the hand. This is a disadvantage for the person who already has stronger flexion (closure) than extension of the hand and needs a better balance of strength. For example, the individual who has had a stroke affecting the upper extremities may experience primitive patterns of muscle return that allow him to close his hand but not open it. The emphasis of activities for that individual should be directed toward increasing extension rather than flexion. This is particularly important for many who have joint disease, such as arthritis, and for whom static positioning only induces further disability. Anyone who does much crocheting or knitting should be encouraged to open and close the hand at frequent intervals to exercise the extensor muscles and improve circulation.
2. Crocheting and knitting are appropriate for the visually limited (some long-term knitters and crocheters can do the work blindfolded), but are not generally suitable for the novice with visual limitations. Larger sized needles and crochet hooks can be employed, and simple straight stitching projects, such as scarves or granny squares, which need not require following written directions, can be done.
3. Straight knitting can be done on a Rake knitting frame (see Appendix B) by a one-handed person if the frame is clamped to a table. Such an arrangement is preferable to one-handed knitting with traditional needles. Although a needle holder is available commercially, it is too awkward for practical use by most one-handers.

Embroidery and crewel are included here, not so much for their physical exercise potential as for their adaptability to the one-handed operator and their usefulness for mental activity and visual planning. Embroidery and crewel require fairly good visual acuity and enough strength to hold onto a needle securely. Since needle placement must be fairly precise, the uncoordinated person might find this activity frustrating, if not almost impossible.

For those with a visual field problem, following a simple line design from a good visual field to an impaired visual field may be a good exercise in compensation, as the participants must learn to turn their heads.

For the person with mild perceptual problems, such as in figure-ground relationships, doing a cross-stitch pattern on a large gingham fabric can be good training. The perceptual ability needed to differentiate top from bottom is most important; it is essential in many self-care abilities (e.g., one must be able to find the collar in contrast to the tail of a shirt or blouse to put on the garment properly).

An obvious advantage of stitchery crafts is the ease with which they can be carried over into the home. They are suitable for a lightly equipped service facility, because they require few supplies. In addition, they offer the potential for innovation in designing one's own project, going beyond the simple stamped kits available.

Needlepoint has many possibilities as a therapeutic medium because it is easily adaptable, with a wide variety of canvas and range of stitching. It has a static component (as for knitting and crocheting), but more frequent opening and closing of the hand is necessary. The craft demands more frequent cutting of threads, which requires additional muscle use for the whole hand. The requirement to place a needle in one hole and bring it up out of another hole makes it necessary to use planning, concentration, eye tracking, and in many instances the mental activity of counting. Because placement of needlepoint can be on the lap, a table, or higher in a clamped frame or stand, it can be adapted easily to individual needs related to exercise requirements and physical limitations. Using longer threads can encourage more active elbow extension if the operator is taught to pull the thread out fully, using a full range of motion.

For the person with joint limitations, the threads can be shorter and the project can be positioned closer to the body. Some people who have neurological disabilities (such as multiple sclerosis) affecting their upper extremities may have better hand control if they keep their arms stabilized close to the body.

For the visually, perceptually, or mentally limited individual, large-hole canvas (such as that normally used for latchhooking—with four holes per inch) can be employed. Something as simple as over-and-under the threads can be done effectively with a simple stripe or block-type pattern, using a heavier yarn or doubling the lighter yarn to cover the canvas.

Since the objective in these activities is independence, it is important to encourage participants to cut thread, thread needles, and start and finish the threads.

For those with limited visual acuity, a major consideration should be to conserve remaining sight. If a person is making frequent errors and appears to be straining visually, it may be due to a poor choice of craft or too small a canvas. It is always wise to try the participant on a sample piece before initiating a full-fledged project, to avoid frustration for both the staff and the participant.

The final finishing process on a project may prove too difficult for some people (e.g., blocking and sewing for backing a pillow). The finished piece can be framed by a family member if the staff or volunteers do not have time for it.

Embroidery and Crewel

The basic stitches in embroidery and crewel appear here in detail. It was felt that these basics would be helpful to a leader (who might lack stitchery experience) in improvising stitches for those with special needs. Also, it provides a dictionary for regular use.

The stitch charts following show some of the differences between embroidery and crewel. The stitches are interchangeable in most cases, depending somewhat on the fabric choice.

The four sample patterns in this section (Figures 13-40 to 13-43) can be enlarged, reduced, or used as shown with embroidery, crewel, or a combination of the two. (See *Enlarging or Reducing a Design,* in this section.)

The fabric used will determine to some extent the weight of thread and size of needle required. Worsted is generally used in crewel work, and cotton and silk floss is used for the lighter, more delicate embroidery stitches.

Figure 13-40 Butterfly Pattern

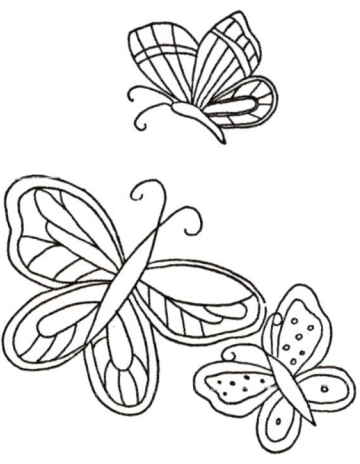

Figure 13-41 Pot Pattern   **Figure 13-42** Eagle Pattern

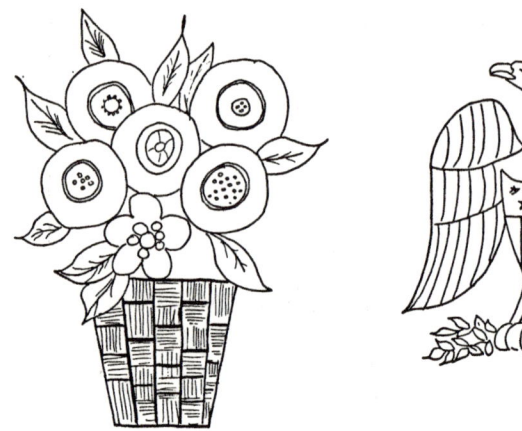
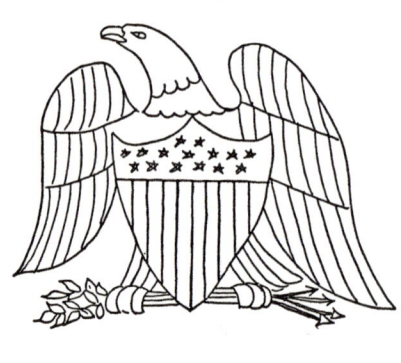

Figure 13-43 Flowering Tree Pattern

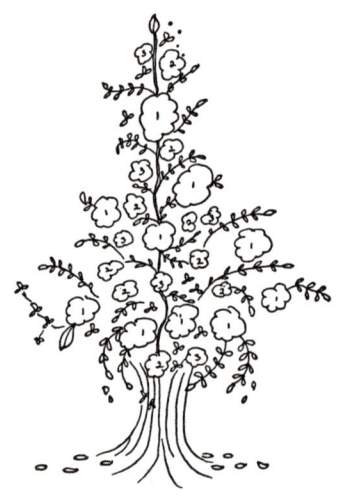

A crewel needle is longer than an embroidery needle and has a longer eye to accommodate the heavier thread or yarn used. For the novice, a sampler is good for beginning. Rows of practice stitches can be made across the fabric, using different colors of yarn or floss to relieve the boredom. Or, a piece of fabric can be marked off into large squares, with different stitches assigned to each square. (See Figure 13-44.)

Figure 13-44 Pattern Marked with Squares

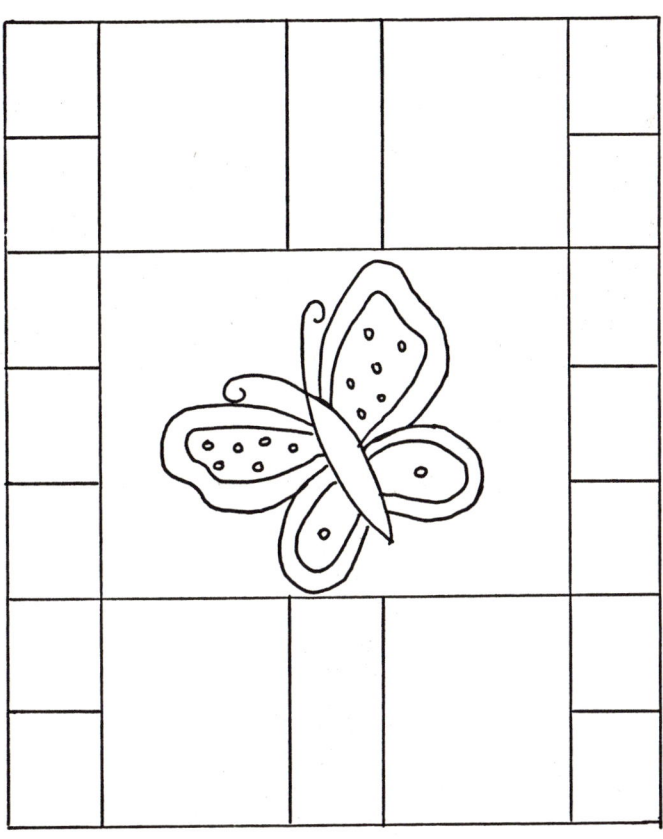

Crewel Stitches

The following illustrations* show some of the basic stitches for crewel work. It is suggested that a sampler be made of these stitches by doing a row or two of each stitch or by making blocks (each with a different stitch) on a piece of fabric and creating a design. The size of the blocks, colors, and stitches can be varied.

Crewel yarn is usually Persian wool (three-strand) or worsted.

---

*Illustrations of crewel stitches here and on the following pages are reproduced by permission of Caron International, 295 Fifth Ave., New York.

Seeding

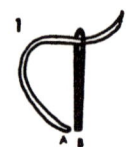 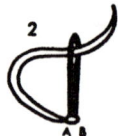 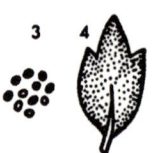

1 & 2. Take two little stitches, one on top of the other, and repeat, scattering them in any direction. 3 & 4. Finished effect.

Stem Stitch

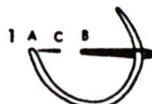 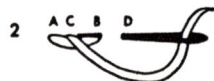 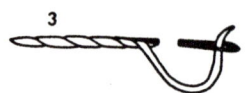

1. Come up at A, go down at B, and up at C. Keep the thread below the needle. 2. Go down at D, up at B (in same hole). 3. Repeat 2. Always keep the thread below the needle.

Split Stitch

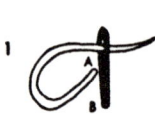 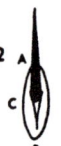 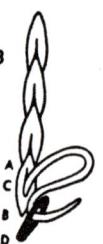

1. Make a straight stitch, A to B. Draw it flat. 2. Come up at C, splitting stitch A-B in the center. 3. Continue, making a smooth row of flat stitches.

Coral Stitch

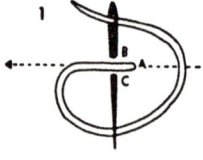 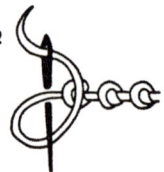

1. Come up at A. Holding the thread flat on the line as shown, go down at B and come up at C, looping the thread under the needle. Pull gently upward to form a loose knot. B-C should be at an exact right angle to the line. 2. Repeat, keeping stitches a "stitch's width" apart.

Craft Projects   133

Satin Stitch

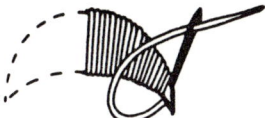

For ease in keeping the angle correct, start in the center of the widest part of the stitch. Come up one side, go down on the other; cross over underneath and come up on the first side again. Repeat, keeping stitches even and side by side.

Satin Stitch with Split Stitch

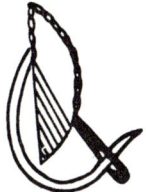

First split stitch around the outline, then satin stitch over the split stitch to form a smooth padded edge. Do not pull too tightly.

Padded Satin Stitch

 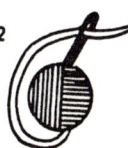

Work satin stitches over the whole shape. Work a second layer of satin stitches over the first, in the opposite direction. (The angle of the final row is always indicated on the design.)

Turkey Work Stitch (Uncut)

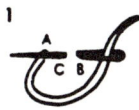 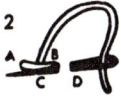 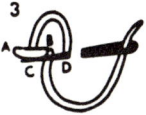 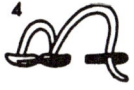 

1. Come up at A, go down at B, then up at C halfway between A and B. Holding the thread below the needle, pull tight. 2. With the thread above the needle, go down at D and come up at B in same hole, leaving a loop. 3 & 4. Repeat, holding the thread below the needle and pulling tight, then above, leaving a loop. Keep the loops even. 5. The line has a finished effect.

Turkey Work Stitch (Cut)

1. Fill in a space with straight rows of Turkey work. Make small stitches and keep the rows close together. Leave loops long enough to trim easily when completed. 2. This gives a finished effect.

Couching Stitch

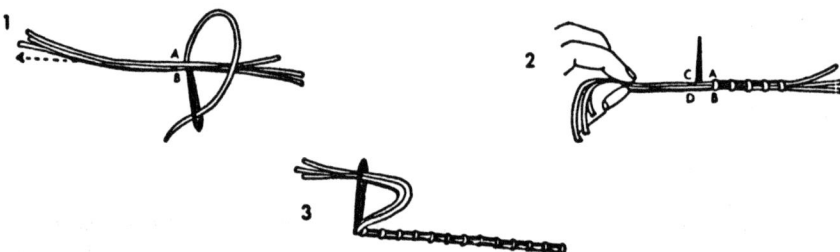

1. Lay the threads along a line. With one thread in the needle, come up at A, down at B. (B is almost in the same hole as A.) 2. Come up at C, about ¼'' from A-B; go down at D. Continue, holding threads taut with the left hand as you sew. 3. At the end of the line, thread the threads into a large-eyed needle and plunge them through the material in the hole made by the last couching stitch. Cut them short (about ¼'') on the reverse side.

Long-and-Short Stitch

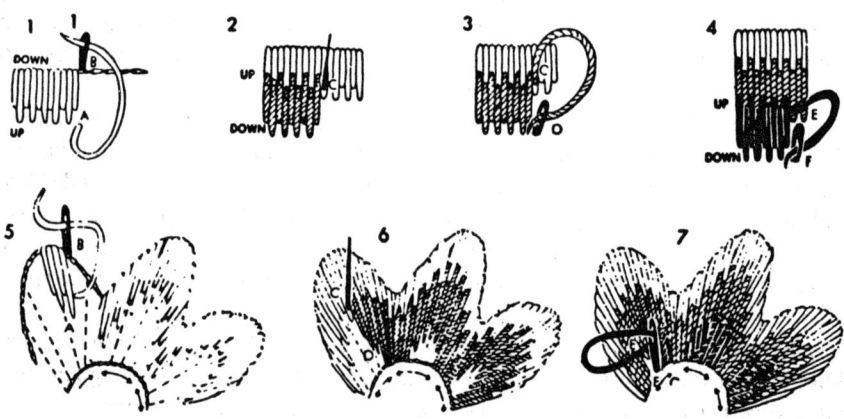

Practice steps 1-4 working vertically, before doing this stitch for the first time. 1. Split stitch around the outline for a neat, padded edge. 1st row: Work straight stitches over the split stitch outline, evenly alternating a long and a short stitch. 2 & 3. 2nd row: Come up at C, splitting the lower third of the stitch in the previous row. Go down at D. Keep all stitches in this and additional rows the same size (the size of the long stitches in the 1st row). 4. Continue, working stitches as shown. 5, 6, & 7. Work the same stitch at gradually changing angles. The exact direction of slant is indicated on the chart or fabric. The preceding illustrations show three blended bands of color, each about the same width.

Embroidery—a Sampler

Materials

1. embroidery hoop
2. scissors
3. embroidery needle (size depends on number of strands of floss used)
4. embroidery floss in assorted colors (comes in six strands, which can be separated)
5. fabric (lightweight cotton, linen, or a synthetic similar to cotton in weave)

Procedure

Select a piece of fabric at least 9″ × 12.″ Allow 1″-1½″ all around for a border. Mark off the area to be worked into blocks of space across the fabric with a ruler and a pencil or felt tip marker.

Choose a few of the stitches from the embroidery stitches chart, Figure 13-45, and work them into the marked-off blocks. Use a variety of colors to make the sampler less boring. Someone new to this might find it advisable to work on a scrap of fabric before blocking off a sampler design.

A suggested sampler, Figure 13-44, blocked off, is shown to stimulate ideas. The size of the sampler can be left to the participant. The butterfly is from Figure 13-40, and can be transferred to fabric by use of dressmaker's carbon placed shiny side down between the fabric and the drawing. (See *Transferring the Design*.) The simple outline stitch and French knots could be a beginning for the butterfly, with other stitches added in the open spaces in the wings and body as they are learned. The blocks around the butterfly will hold a variety of stitches.

The seeding stitch in the crewel stitchery chart can be substituted for the French knot (which requires the use of two hands). Place three or four seeding stitches close together in place of each French knot; the effect will be similar.

Figure 13-45 Embroidery Stitches

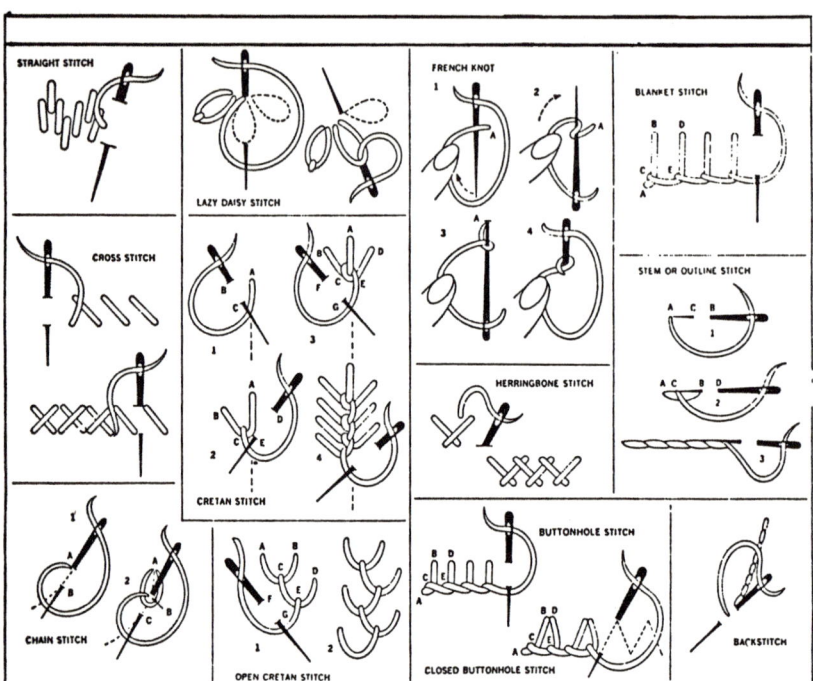

Variations

- luncheon cloths with corner and center motifs
- placemats and napkins
- pillowcase border designs
- designs on ready-made blouses, jeans, or jackets
- kits with pre-stamped designs (see Appendix C)

Adaptations for Embroidery and Crewel Work

- Embroidery hoops or frames can be clamped to the table. The special needle threader described in this section will enable the one-handed person to become independent in needle threading.

- For those with limited concentration power, designs and stitches can be simplified.
- See Appendix B for additional assistive equipment.
- Pre-stamped embroidery kits can be used. For beginners, large, simple designs are best. (See list of suppliers, Appendix C, for the source for sampler kits.)

Crewel—a Sampler

Materials

1. embroidery hoop
2. scissors
3. crewel needle (size depends on weight of wool used)
4. crewel yarn or worsted (comes in three strands, which can be separated)
5. fabric (linen or other heavier weight material)

Procedure

The procedure is the same as for the embroidery sampler. The sampler design, Figure 13-44, can be used, but the heavier fabric and crewel stitches will produce a different look. For example, the cut Turkey work stitch can be used for the body of the butterfly, giving it a fuzzy, three-dimensional effect.

Variations

The heavier fabric used for crewel work lends itself well to making belts (which can be lined), place mats, wall hangings, and pillows. Figure 13-43 can be a combination of three different sizes of flowers, made on a flower loom widely available in variety stores, and crewel stitches. Enlarge the drawing (see *Enlarging or Reducing a Design*) to 16" × 24," and work on a natural or contrasting background of linen, Indianhead, or fine burlap. Slip a dowel stick through the top hem for a wall hanging, or mat and frame as you would a picture.

Enlarging or Reducing a Design

Materials

1. tracing paper
2. kraft or other heavy paper

3. ruler
4. fine-line black pen
5. blunt tool and carbon if design is to be transferred directly to fabric (see *Transferring the Design*)

Procedure
1. On tracing paper, make a grid of small squares, 1″ or ½.″ Begin by drawing a horizontal and a vertical line intersecting at the top lefthand corner to form a right angle.

2. Mark off the squares and number them from left to right and top to bottom.

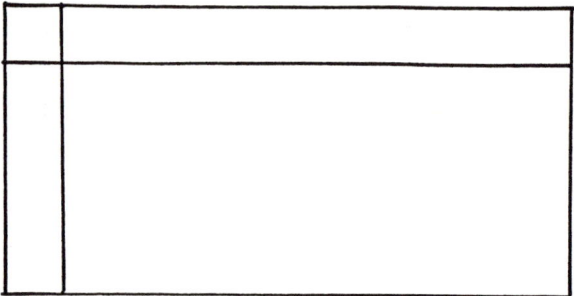

3. Place the grid over the design to be enlarged and trace the design with a fine black pen. Remove the grid from the design.
4. Make a corresponding grid of large squares on kraft paper to represent the size of the final drawing; e.g., if the small grid has ½″ squares and the design is to be enlarged to twice the size of the original, the squares on the large grid should be 1.″ (See Figures 13-46 through 13-49. To reduce a design, follow the procedure in reverse.)

Craft Projects 139

Figure 13-46 Small Design to Be Enlarged

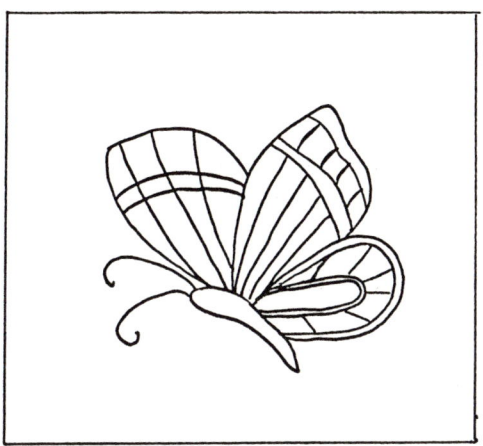

Figure 13-47 Tracing Paper over Design

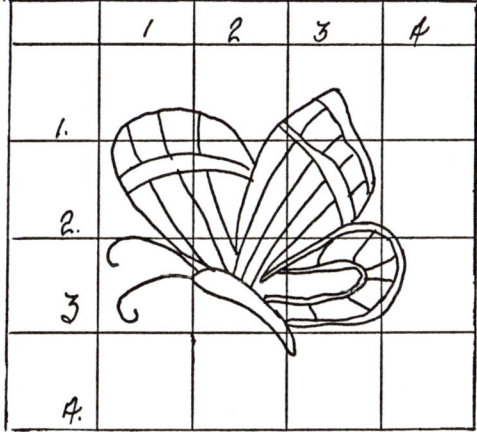

Figure 13-48 Large Grid on Heavy Paper

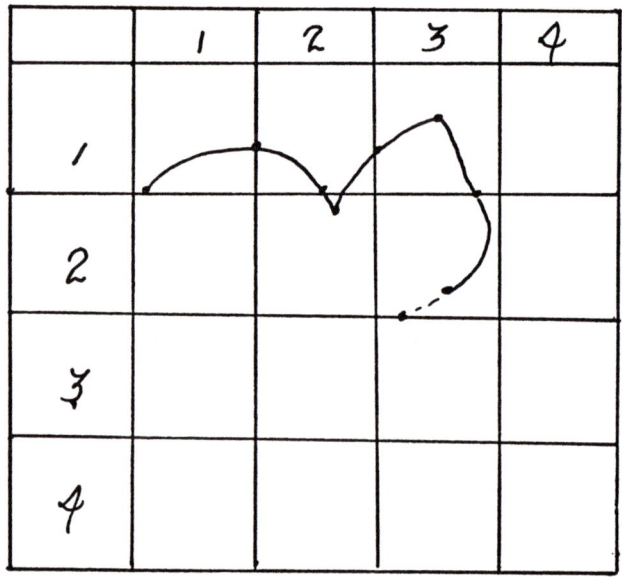

Figure 13-49 Completed Enlargement

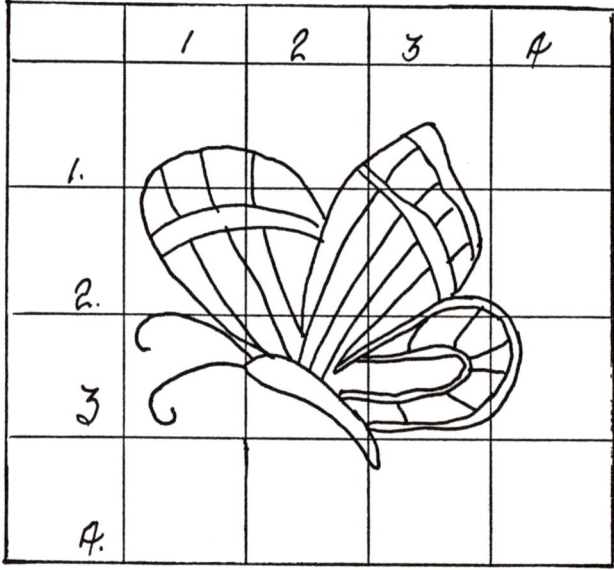

Transferring the Design

Use dressmaker's carbon to transfer designs to fabric. Place the carbon shiny side down on the fabric and the design face up on the carbon. Trace the design, checking occasionally to see if carbon lines are transferring to the fabric. Work from top to bottom to avoid smudging.

To transfer a design onto a loose-weave fabric which will not receive carbon markings, place the design on top of the fabric and use a heavy needle to make pin pricks along the lines of the drawing. Then rub or sprinkle powdered chalk on the design. The chalk will seep through the holes and become a guide for marking with a waterproof marker. Check occasionally to see if the chalk is seeping through and transferring the design clearly enough for later marking.

To transfer a design to needlepoint canvas, place the canvas over the design and copy the design onto the canvas with a waterproof marker. Special markers are available, in colors, so a design can also be "painted" in if desired. Note: The lines on the design to be placed under the canvas for tracing will have to be very dark for good visibility through the mesh.

A two- or three-inch margin should be left all around the design for finishing, and to allow for taping the edges before working, as described in the needlepoint project, following.

Needlepoint and Bargello

Needlepoint and Bargello stitches are worked over a canvas mesh which is available in a range of sizes classified by the number of holes per inch: No. 10 mesh, No. 12 mesh, etc. Canvas comes in two basic types: mono, which has single threads spaced the same distance apart, and duo, which has two pairs of threads.

No. 10 mesh canvas (with 10 holes per inch) is a good size for most beginners. It has enough space between the threads for good visibility for those with slight visual problems, and has the advantage of working up quickly for people limited to the use of one hand or those with limited concentration.

A three-strand acrylic yarn should be used, with a No. 18 needle. Knitting worsted can be used, but has too much elasticity to provide the proper tension.

The proper length of the yarn can be determined by the reach desired for each participant if the project is being used for therapy. Otherwise, an 18″ to 24″ length of yarn should be used. Longer lengths tend to get "nubby" from being pulled through the holes.

Small projects, such as eyeglasses cases, small pillows, and pin cushions, are suggested as beginning projects.

Needlepoint canvas is sold by the yard and number of holes per inch. For fine needlepoint, use a No. 14 mesh canvas, with 2 strands of Persian wool and a No. 20 needle. For medium-weight work, use a No. 12 mesh canvas, with 2 strands of

Persian wool and a No. 18 needle. For coarse-weight work, use a No. 10 mesh canvas, with 3 strands of Persian wool and a No. 18 needle. (Persian wool is mentioned here as a standard against which to compare acrylic or other yarn weights used.)

"No-frame" rug canvas is of heavier quality and preferable when a wood frame is not to be used.

The most practical yarn is Persian wool because it is made of three easily separated strands, thus permitting the use of all three strands, two strands, or a single strand of yarn.

Tapestry yarn is a thicker single strand made to fit a specific canvas size; different brands vary in thickness.

Acrylic and worsted yarns also may be used.

Crewel yarn (a thin single strand yarn) or thread may be introduced to highlight the work.

The proper weight of yarn must be chosen so that canvas threads are not visible when the work is completed.

Instructions for needlepoint and Bargello stitches and projects can be found in any of the many books listed in the bibliography. One or two sessions at a local craft center will pay dividends for the leader who wishes to use this craft but is unfamiliar with it. The simple project given here (an eyeglasses case) introduces the basic stitches in needlepoint and Bargello.

Projects chosen will depend on the ability of the person learning the skill. Always start with a small, simple design or pattern so that the quick completion of the project will act as a motivator.

Adaptations for Those with the Use of Only One Hand

After covering the edge of the canvas with masking tape, tack through taped canvas to a wooden frame. Anchor the frame with a C-clamp, or utilize the embroidery frame listed in Appendix B or the Sit-On Stitchery frame. Use also the special needle threader for one-handed sewing shown in this section.

Adaptations for Those with Limited Vision

- Use yarn in strong contrasting colors.
- Use special self-threading yarn threader. (See Appendix B.)
- Use large-mesh canvas (No. 5 mesh) and heavier yarns.
- Note that straight needlepoint, such as the half-cross stitch or the Continental stitch, is easier than the basket-weave stitch.
- If the participant has visual field limitations, be sure the work is positioned in the good visual field. It may be helpful for the instructor to put in one line of needlepoint (particularly in Bargello) as a guide.

Adaptations for Those Limited in Shoulder Strength or Range of Motion

The participant can work at lap level. The sit-on frame, listed in Appendix B, is useful here.

Bargello

Bargello is done entirely with one simple upright (vertical) stitch, varied only by the number of threads over which it is worked. Figure 13-50 shows a basic stitch (the zig-zag) covering four threads of canvas.

Anchoring the yarn to start Bargello is the same as for starting needlepoint. If the waste knot is used, be sure it is cut off after the beginning stitches are secure. (See Figure 13-57.)

End a length of yarn by weaving it through three or four stitches at the back of the work. Cut off the excess yarn.

It is important to select a yarn suitable to the canvas used. It must be of the proper weight (thickness) to cover the mesh threads completely. The straight up and down stitches of Bargello, which lie between the threads, will accommodate a heavier yarn than needlepoint stitches, which lie over intersections of the threads.

Figure 13-50 Zig-Zag Pattern

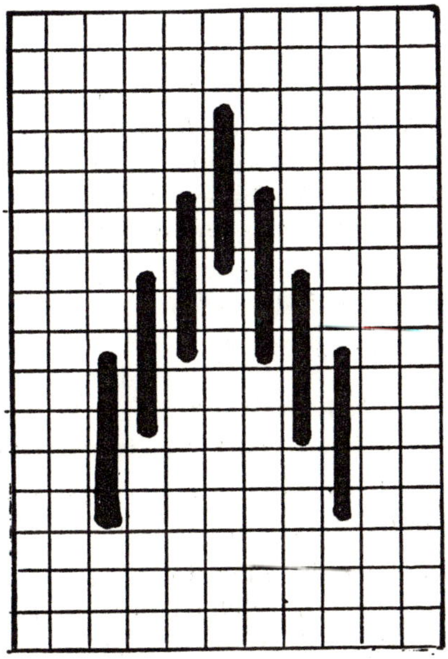

Tapestry needles are used for Bargello and should be sized to pass through the canvas mesh with ease:

- No. 18 needle for No. 10 mesh canvas
- No. 20 needle for No. 12 or 13 mesh canvas
- No. 22 needle for No. 14 or 16 mesh canvas

The pattern given here for an eyeglasses case uses the 4-2 step (Figure 13-53) for the flame or zig-zag stitch (Figure 13-50), and calls for three colors of yarn. The simplicity of the Bargello embroidery stitch calls for shading or contrast, or both, in yarn selection.

Bargello Eyeglasses Case

Materials

1. No. 10 canvas, 7" × 7"
2. masking tape, 1" wide
3. 4-strand Orylon-acrylic yarn, 3 colors
4. tapestry needle, No. 18
5. scissors
6. ruler
7. felt or other soft fabric for lining
8. sewing needle and thread

Procedure

Determine the proper canvas size by laying the glasses on the canvas, folding it over them, and adding 1½" to the length and width for finishing.

Cut the canvas (7" × 7" in this example) and cover the edges with masking tape. (1" tape will provide a good margin for finishing the edges.) The working area the stitches will cover is now 6½" × 6½".

Find the center of the working area by folding the canvas in half, then in half again; or, draw lines diagonally from corner to corner. Where the two lines meet, mark the center with a cross to use as a guide in placing the design. (See Figure 13-51.)

Use color A for the first row across the canvas. The design is centered on the canvas. (See Figure 13-52.) One half is worked from the center of the canvas to the right edge, and the other half from the center to the left edge. Figure 13-53 shows how the 4-2 step is worked: Come up over four threads and down under two threads. (Come up at odd numbers, go down at even.)

Figure 13-51 Marking the Center

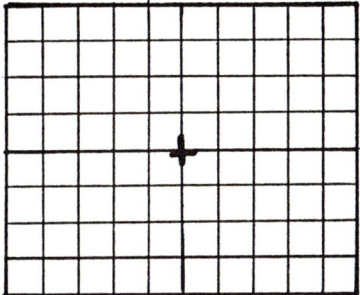 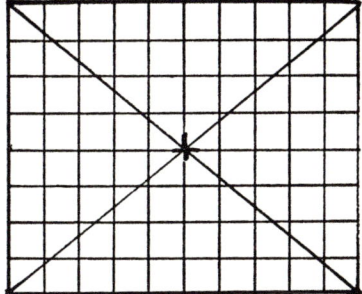

Figure 13-52 Asterisk Marks Center Stitch (Zig-Zag Pattern)

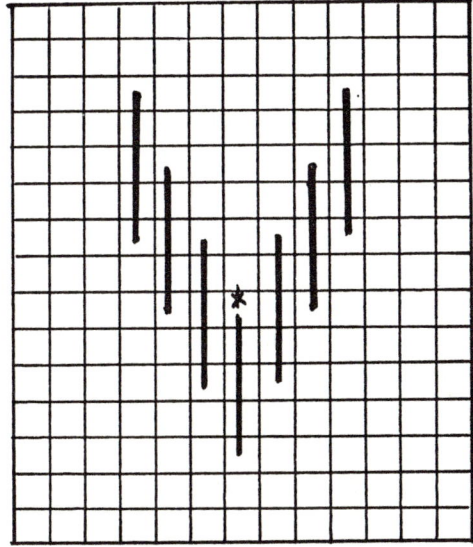

This completes the base (or key) row, which is used as a guide for the rest of the work. With color B, starting at the left of the canvas, come up four holes below the first stitch at the edge, over four threads, and down into the space taken up by the first stitch. Continue in the pattern to the right edge of the canvas with color B, then repeat with color C for the third row. (Stitches can be worked back and forth across the canvas, if desired.) Colors A, B, and C will now be repeated down to the bottom line of the working area. Figure 13-54 shows a completed pattern and indicates the place of the three colors in the design.

Figure 13-53 4-2 Step (up at 1, down at 2, etc.)

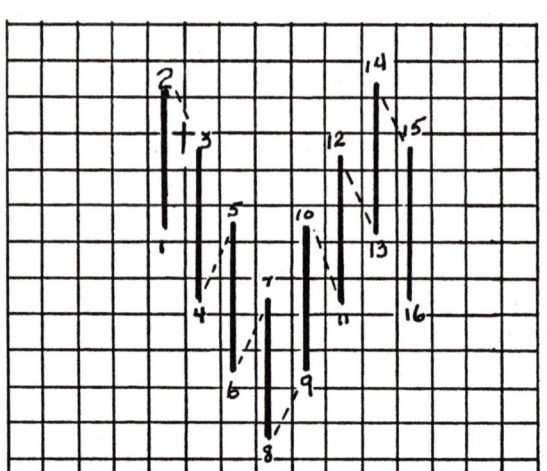

Figure 13-54 Three-Color Zig-Zag Pattern

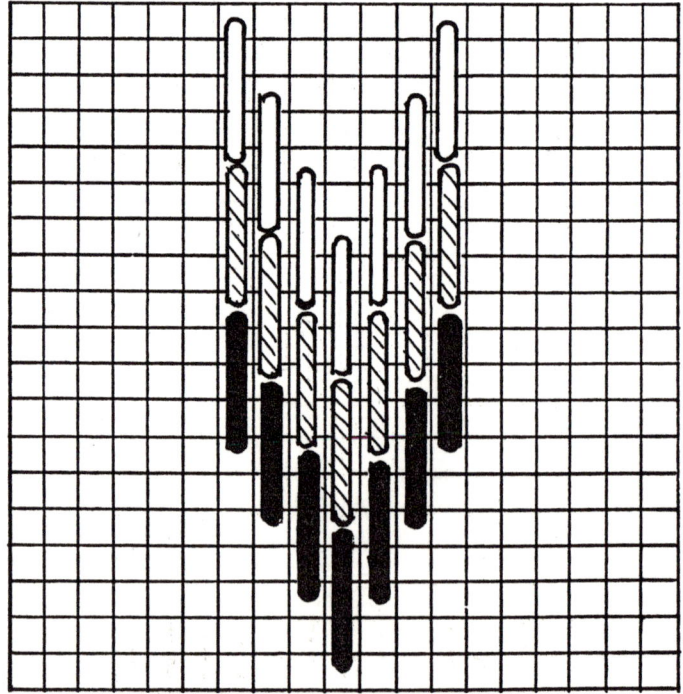

Craft Projects 147

Compensating Stitches. There will be open spaces of two threads in the mesh when the bottom line is reached. Fill in these spaces with the color called for in the design, keeping the color scheme with these smaller stitches. All threads in the canvas working area must be covered. Figure 13-55 shows compensating stitches at the bottom of the work.

When the bottom half of the canvas has been stitched, turn the work around so the bottom becomes the top. Start with color B beneath the base row (which was color A) at the left side of the canvas, and follow the color scheme set up for the beginning work—base row A, second row B, third row C—then repeat.

When the lower section is completed, the pattern for the top and bottom should end at the same place in the design. Use compensating stitches to finish off. The sides of the design should be even since there was a built-in control in setting up the base row across the canvas.

Figure 13-55 Compensating Stitches

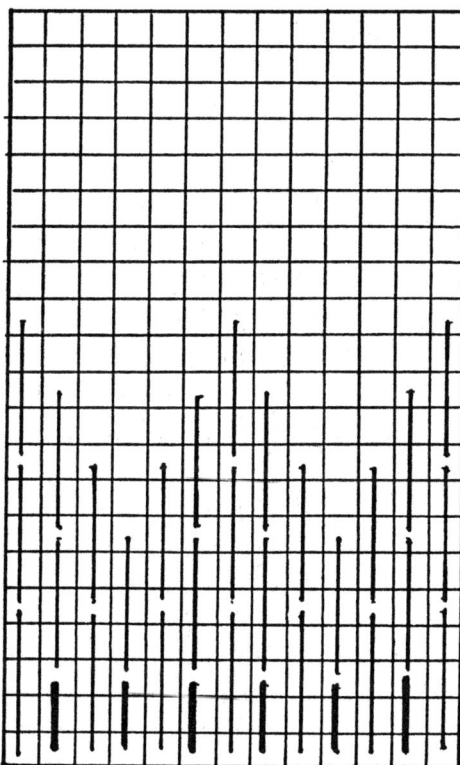

The Lining. Working with the finished piece open, cover what will be the open end of the eyeglasses case with a blanket stitch (Figure 13-45) or a single cordovan stitch (Figure 13-63), stitching over the tape. Run the yarn ends through the stitches to hide them.

With the work still open, line it by tacking a piece of light fabric or felt (felt works well, because it does not need hemming) to the edges of the wrong side of the work. Do not cover the tape. Caution: When pinning the lining in place prior to sewing, leave enough overlap to allow for folding the case in half.

When the lining is stitched in place, fold the case in half and finish the side and bottom by covering the tape with a buttonhole stitch (Figure 13-45) or single cordovan stitch, as was done for the opening. Cut the corners of the canvas slightly before stitching to give a nicer finish. (The rounded corner is easier to cover with multiple stitches.)

Variations

- Use one of the needlepoint stitches with variegated yarn, which will create its own pattern.
- Reduce the size of the pattern and make a pincushion.
- Enlarge the size and make a pillow.
- Experiment with different colors, metallic threads, and different stitch lengths in Bargello.
- Try kits for different size projects (available at craft and department stores). (See Appendix C for a list of craft kit suppliers.)

Adaptations

See *Adaptations* in the *Needlepoint and Bargello* Section.

Needlepoint

Beginning a Needlepoint Piece

Work needlepoint stitches at an angle across the mesh of the canvas where the vertical and horizontal lines cross. (See Figure 13-56.)

Figure 13-56
Needlepoint Stitches

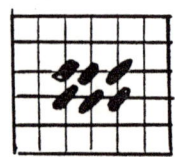

Anchoring the Yarn

Tie a knot in the yarn. (See *Tying a Knot with One Hand.*) Insert the needle from the front of the canvas three or four holes from the beginning of your work. After the first three or four stitches have covered the yarn, cut off the knot and continue across the canvas. (This is the waste knot. See Figure 13-57.) Or, leave a 1" tail of yarn at the back of the canvas, hold it in place in the direction of your work, and cover it as you stitch.

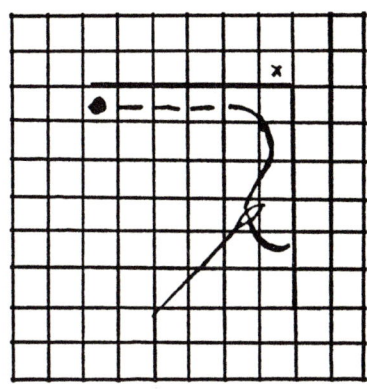

Figure 13-57 The Waste Knot

For the person with a hand disability, a length of yarn (1" to 2") can be left dangling at the back of the work. After the work is completed, secure the loose ends with a touch of white glue, diluted half and half, and cut off the excess yarn.

Ending a Length of Yarn

With the needle at the back of the work, weave back through three or four stitches of finished work. Cut off the excess yarn.

Starting a New Length of Yarn

Use one of the three methods described in *Anchoring the Yarn.*

Blocking the Needlepoint

Dampen the finished needlepoint piece and place it right-side-down on a wooden board. Square up the corners and tack the sides, top, and bottom securely to the board with rustproof tacks. Place the tacks about 1" apart. (Some stretching may be needed to line up the vertical and horizontal mesh of the canvas.) Leave the canvas on the board for 24 hours. Remove it from the board and repeat the process if necessary.

The Half-Cross Stitch

This stitch is used for pillows, wall hangings, and other articles that will not receive heavy wear. It requires less yarn than the Continental or basket-weave stitches. (See Figure 13-58.) Work from left to right. Bring the needle up at 1, down at 2, up at 3, down at 4, etc., across the row. At the end of the row, put the

Figure 13-58 The Half-Cross Stitch

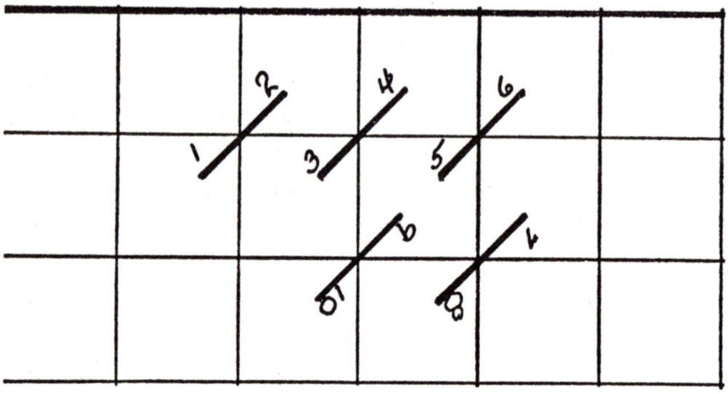

needle down at 6, turn the canvas, bring the needle up at 7 and down at 8, and continue across the row. (Once the stitch has been learned by doing a few practice rows, it is not necessary to turn the canvas after each row.)

The Continental Stitch

This stitch is best for outlining and filling in small areas, because it distorts the canvas. For large pieces, blocking is necessary. However, it is a popular stitch with beginners. (See Figure 13-59.) Work from right to left. Bring the needle up at 1, down at 2, up at 3, and down at 4. Continue across the row. At the end of the row, put the needle down at 10. Turn the canvas around, bring the needle up at 11, down at 12, and continue across the row as before. Always work from right to left, turning the work at the end of each row. (The alternative to turning the canvas upside down at the end of each row is to have the needle come up at 12, down at 11, up at 14, down at 13, etc.)

Figure 13-59 The Continental Stitch

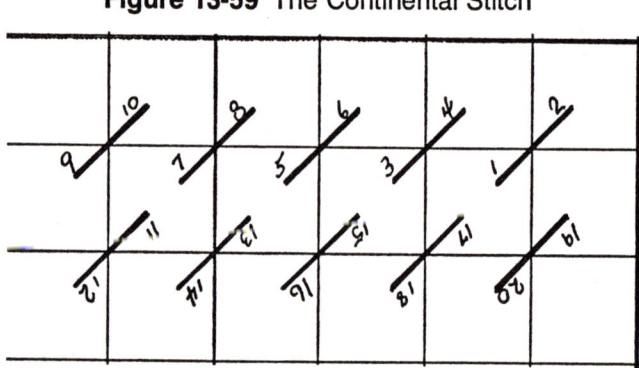

The Basket-Weave Stitch

This stitch is good for backgrounds and large areas of color, because it causes little distortion of the canvas. It may be worked without turning the canvas. (See Figure 13-60.) Because this stitch has a basket-weave padded back, it is especially good for chairs, footstools, and other much used furniture. It requires a minimum of blocking. Begin at the upper right corner. Come up at 1, down at 2, etc., through 8. Increase one stitch each side until the maximum width is obtained. Once the pattern is established, change in the canvas area to be covered can be made by continuing the established row. The basket-weave stitch is difficult to learn, but is shown here to complete the trio of "tent" stitches (the others are the half-cross and the Continental). These three stitches look alike on the front of the canvas but each has its own characteristics and advantages because of the way the back of the canvas receives the yarn, the extent of canvas distortion, and the amount of yarn used.

Figure 13-60 The Basket-Weave Stitch

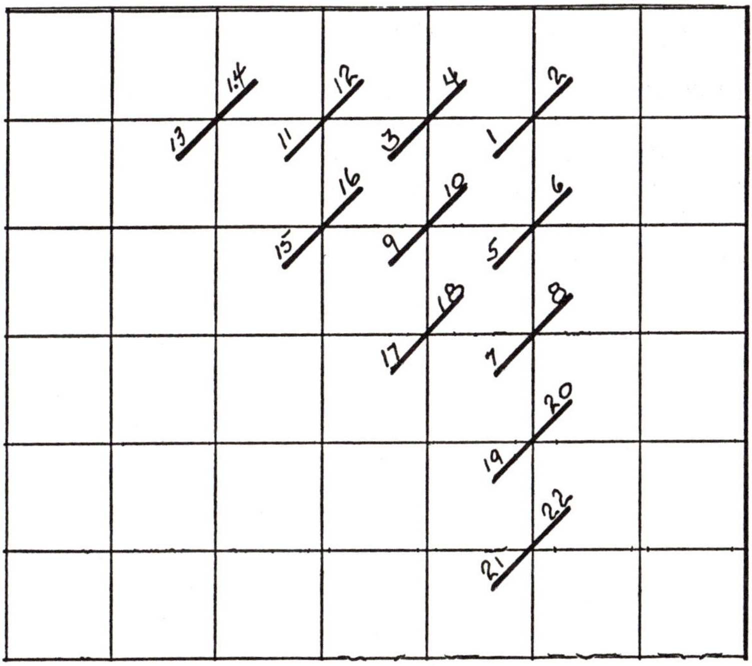

Needlepoint Eyeglasses Case

Materials

Use the same materials as called for in the Bargello project.

Procedure

Cut the canvas (7″ × 7″, for example) and cover the edges with masking tape. (1″ tape will provide a good margin for finishing the edges.) The working area the stitches will cover is 6½″ × 6½.″

Follow the directions for either the half-cross stitch (Figure 13-58) or the Continental stitch (Figure 13-59) to fill the working area.

Mark a geometric design on the canvas mesh with a waterproof marker. Choose three colors for the design. Work the design area first, then fill in the background color. Follow the directions for the lining described for the *Bargello Eyeglasses Case*. Or, remove the masking tape, turn the canvas edges to the wrong side of the work, fold the case in half, and stitch the bottom and side seams. Insert a lining that has been seamed on the bottom and one side. Then stitch the lining to the open end of the case (using small stitches so they will not be snagged when the case is used). Hem the top of the lining (unless felt is used).

Variation

Use a variegated yarn which contains multiple colors and shades. This will create its own design.

Making a One-Handed Needle Threader*

Materials

1. hammer
2. 4 nails 1½″ or 2″ long
3. scissors
4. ¾″ pine, 4½″ × 6,″ for base
5. felt strip for bottom of base, 4½″ × 6″
6. felt strip for top of base, 4½″ × 2″

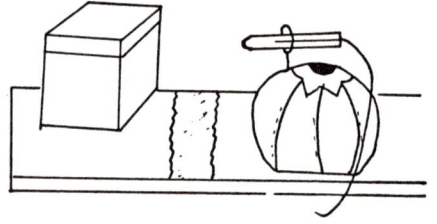

---

*The special needle threader presented here was designed by Ann Krieger, a volunteer at Burke Rehabilitation Center's Day Hospital.

7. small box with easy-to-lift off lid to hold threader tubes and needles
8. clear plastic straws, cut and shaped as shown
9. white glue
10. blunt tapestry needles
11. purchased pincushion (firm and solid)

Procedure

Sand and shellac the base. Let it dry thoroughly.

Glue, then nail, the pincushion to one end of the wood base. The four nails will anchor it securely.

Glue the small box on the other end of the wood base. Cut and glue on the felt strips for the bottom and top of the base. (Pinking shears give a nice finish for the top strip.) Anchor the finished base to the table with a C-clamp if desired. The top strip of felt protects the base from clamp marks; the bottom strip protects the table surface and keeps the base from sliding if a C-clamp is not used.

Cut the plastic straws into 2'' or 2½'' lengths. Squeeze a straw at one end and pass it through the eye of a tapestry needle several times, but allow the straw to retain its shape; do not flatten. The end of the straw that went through the needle's eye first is the end to shape.

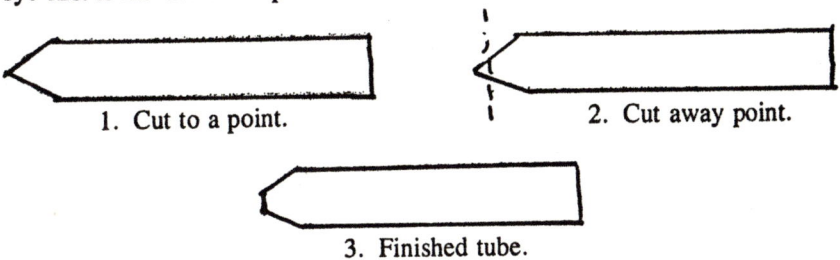

1. Cut to a point. 2. Cut away point.

3. Finished tube.

The tubes can be used until they become too flat and prevent feeding of the yarn into the tube.

Using the Needle Threader

1. Insert a tapestry needle more than halfway into the pincushion.
2. Push a plastic tube into the eye of the needle until it is firmly held.
3. Insert the yarn into the tube.
4. Push, then pull, the tube through the needle's eye so that the yarn comes with it.

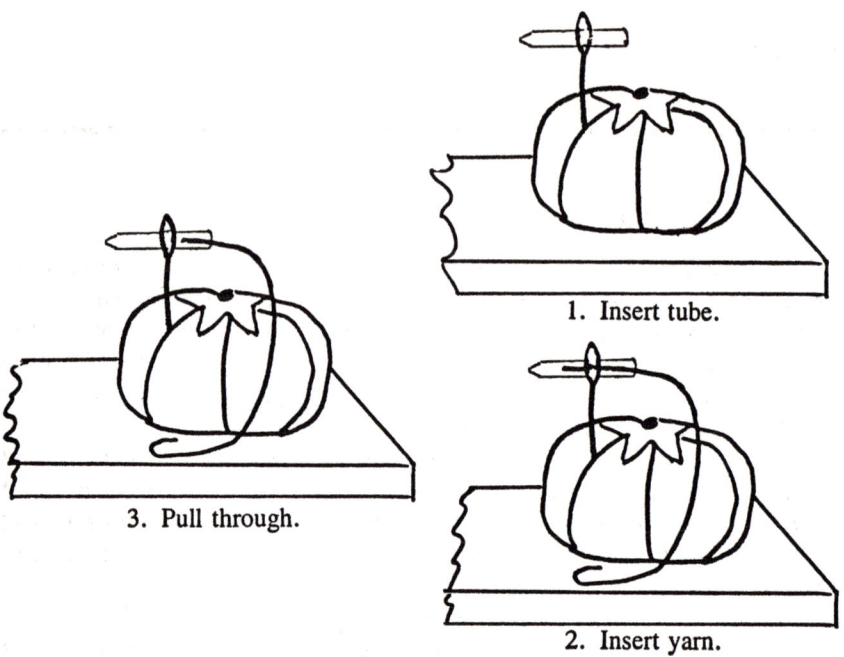

1. Insert tube.
2. Insert yarn.
3. Pull through.

Tying a Knot With One Hand

Push two corsage pins into the pincushion with the points close together but the tops about an inch apart.

After the needle has been threaded, secure the end of the yarn to be knotted close to the base of the two corsage pins with a small plastic-headed pin. Push the pin into the yarn end until just the pin head shows.

Hold the threaded needle, twist the yarn counterclockwise around the upright corsage pins, and return to the left of the small plastic-headed pin. Push the needle under and up through the loop thus formed. Pull the yarn taut at the base of the two corsage pins to form a knot, then remove the small pin to release the yarn end. Remove the corsage pins to free the knot.

Left-handed sewers should follow the directions in reverse, going clockwise after the yarn end is anchored into the pincushion.

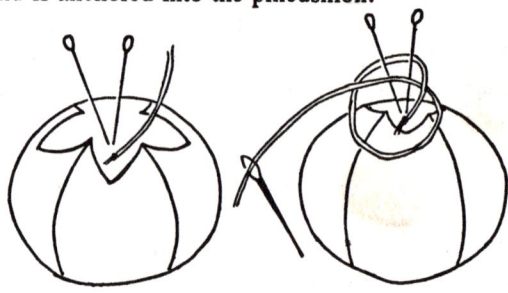

LEATHER LACING

Therapeutic Implications

Leatherwork encompasses a variety of techniques and skills that can add interest to an activity program. It has a broad appeal, even for men who may reject other activities. Basically, leather projects may be stamped, carved or laced to make them into attractive articles. As most of these techniques are well covered in leathercraft books, included here are only a few basic lacing projects that can be used by participants with chronic disabilities.

Stamping and carving of leather are difficult for someone with the use of only one hand, but they are good exercises for strengthening the prehension and wrist muscles where mild impairment exists. The pounding involved with stamping tools can be used to vent frustration for some people. Punching holes for leather lacing is a good exercise for increasing grasp strength.

Leather lacing can be done with pre-cut kits and punched with very little equipment. Preparing projects from raw leather requires good use of both hands as well as good vision.

Pre-cut link belts can be used by the visually limited, and their contrasting texture helps develop a sense of touch. The link belts can be held in a vise for the one-handed person.

Suggestions on Lacing

1. Except for those with obvious skill in this craft, it is best to start on a small project with a simple stitch, such as the whipstitch or single cordovan.
2. For those with tightness in the shoulders or elbows, place the work in a table vise. (It can be put on an adjustable table to elevate it higher than a normal table top.) Encourage participants to pull the lace tight, using elbow extension.
3. Always have people work from left to right with the outside of the work facing them, so that the stitches will lie flatter. Instructors should be consistent in teaching this technique to avoid confusing the participants.
4. The shorter the piece of lace, the less chance for twists. (This is especially important for a confused, visually limited, or uncoordinated person.)

    In measuring the amount of lace, allow 3½ times around the area to be laced for the whipstitch, 5½ times around for the single cordovan, and 7½ times around for the double cordovan.
5. Leather lacing (unlike plastic lacing) has definite right and wrong sides, making it easier to get out twists; also, it is easier to pull tight.

6. If the participant has a visual problem, contrasting color of lace and work is advantageous, as is having larger holes punched. If there is a visual field problem, be sure the work is placed in the good visual field.
7. Preassembling the work may be necessary for some. It is particularly helpful to tie the corners together to make sure the holes are lined up (or the project can be glued together with rubber cement to ease handling).
8. A lacing needle makes it easier to get the lace through the holes, or an awl can be used to enlarge the holes.
9. Those with a usable but weak hand should be encouraged to pull out the lace with this hand, even if they lack the control or strength to get the needle in.

The Single Whipstitch

Figure 13-61 Single Whipstitch.

To accomplish the whipstitch, start by putting the needle through a hole from front to back and pull the lacing through the hole until almost to the end. Hold about an inch of the end under the thumb before it is pulled through. Put the needle through the next hole (do not twist the lacing), pull the lacing through, and continue. (See Figure 13-61.)*

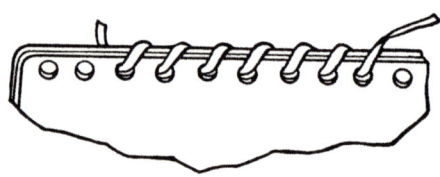

When the end of a lace is reached: If two thicknesses of leather are being laced, put the needle through the hole in the first layer of leather, then down between the layers. Start the new lace by putting the needle between the two layers, then through the hole of the second layer of leather toward the back, then continue lacing. The two ends between the layers can be cut off at about 1″ and glued along the edge. If just one piece of leather is being laced, the ends are run under the lacing for about an inch on the underside, or each piece to be joined can be skived (pared), then glued together.

Ending a single whipstitch: Continue lacing until all the holes are laced. This brings the working end right up to the 1″ end left at the beginning. Pull the beginning end down, out of the hole in the first layer of lacing, and down between the layers of leather. (See Figure 13-62.) Put the working end through the hole in the first layer of leather and then down between the layers.

---

*Figures 13-61 through 13-69 are from TM8-290, *Craft Techniques in Occupational Therapy*, by permission of the Office of the Surgeon General, Department of the Army.

Craft Projects   157

Figure 13-62 Splicing Single Whipstitch.

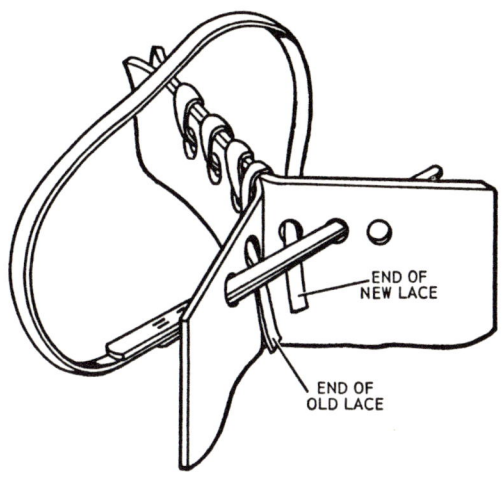

Figure 13-63 The Single Cordovan

Step 1. To start the lacing, insert the working end of the lacing into the starting hole from front to back. Pull it through the hole except for about 1 inch, which is held down on the back so it forms a loop.

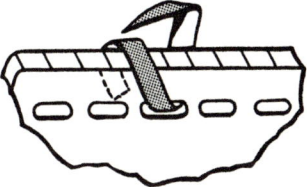

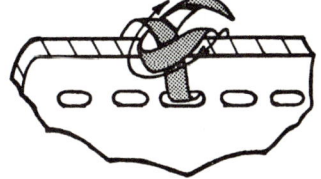

Step 2. Take the working end of the lacing from the back of the piece, bring it toward the front and put it under the loop.

Step 3. Bring the working end of the lacing from the back to the front and insert it into the second hole and pull the lacing through.

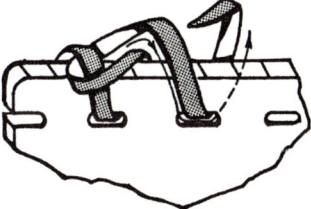

Figure 13-63 continued

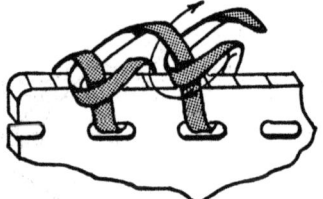

Step 4. Next bring the working end from the back to the front and insert it under the single strand of the loop made by the lacing in Step 3.

Step 5. Repeat Steps 3 and 4 through the hole and under the loop until the last stitch is completed in the hole next to the starting hole.

Figure 13-64

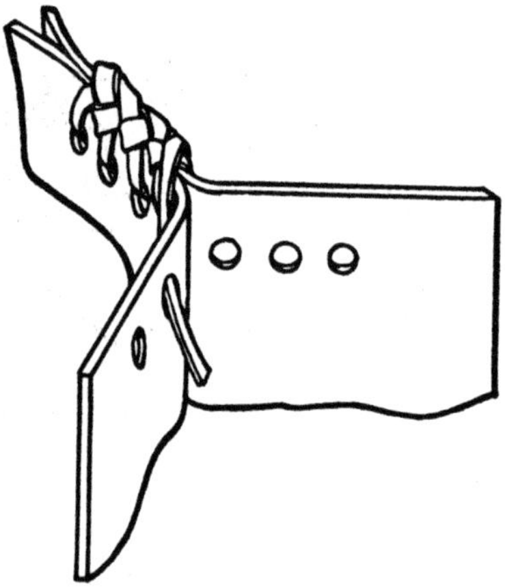

Step 1. Bring the working end of the lacing from the back to the front and insert it through the hole of the top layer of leather, then down between the two leathers.

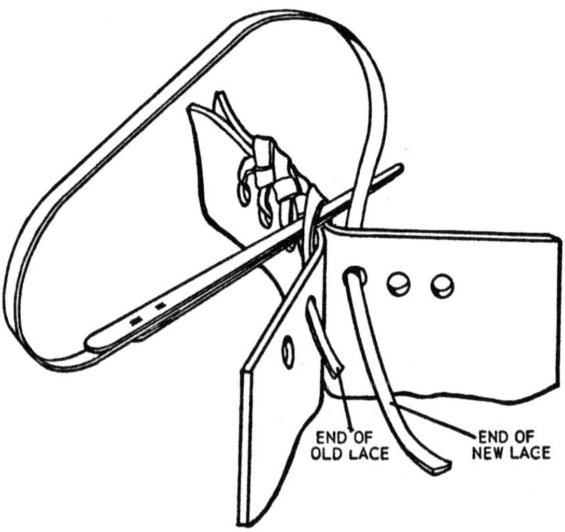

Step 2. Start the new piece by putting it up between the layers of leather, through the hole in the bottom piece of leather and then around the front and under the loop made by the last piece of lacing. Continue lacing.

END OF OLD LACE   END OF NEW LACE

Craft Projects   159

Figure 13-65

Step 1. Lace up to the starting hole as illustrated.

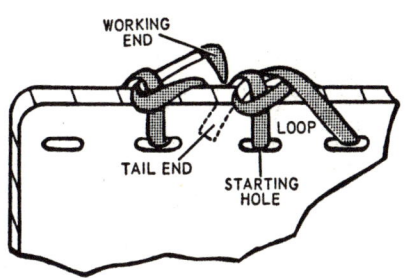

Step 2. Pull the 1-inch tail out of the loop at the first starting hole, and insert the working end of the lacing through this loop. Be sure to maintain the original position of the loop.

Step 3. Pull the tail end of the lacing out of the hole in the top layer of leather and down between the two layers.

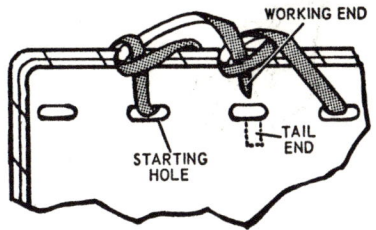

Step 4. Complete by putting the working end through the hole in the top layer of leather and down between the two layers of leather. Cut the ends to about 1 inch and glue down.

Figure 13-66

Step 1. Insert the working end of the lace through the starting hole. Leave about a 1" tail. Bend this tail over so it forms a loop and hold it in place with the hand that is holding the project.

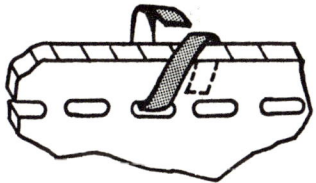

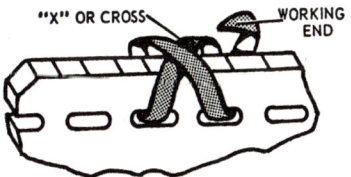

Step 2. Bring the working end of the lace over this loop and through the next hole. The loops cross over one another forming the X.

Figure 13-66 continued

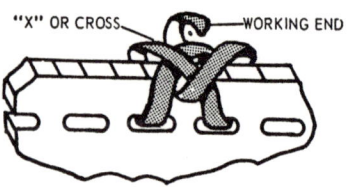

Step 3. Bring the working end of the lace over and back under this X. Tighten this stitch by pulling the lace.

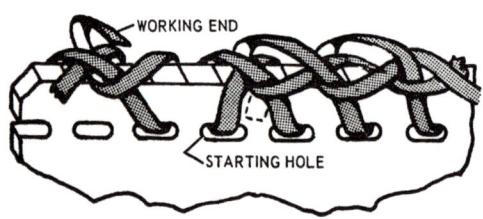

Step 4. Repeat through the hole and under the cross until the last stitch is completed in the hole next to the starting hole.

Figure 13-67

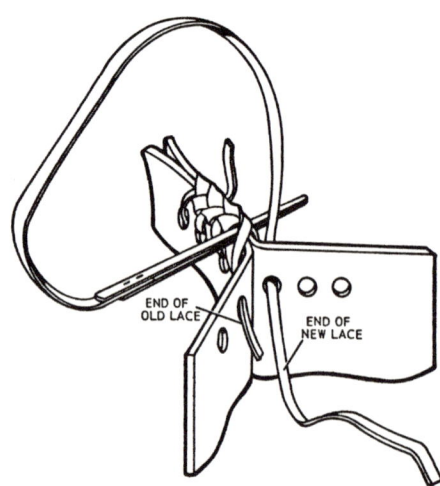

Figure 13-68

Step 1. Pull the tail completely out of the starting stitch and hole.

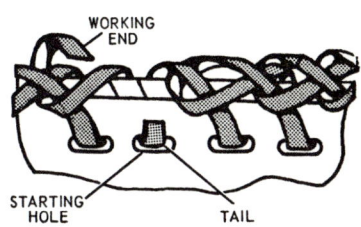

Step 2. Pull the tail out of the loop, leaving the loop free and the tail hanging loosely. Make sure the loop maintains the same position as it did in the stitch.

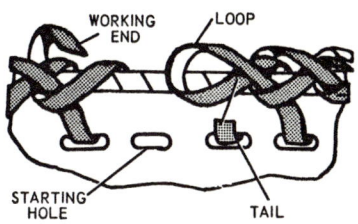

Step 3. Bring the working end of the lacing through the starting hole which is free.

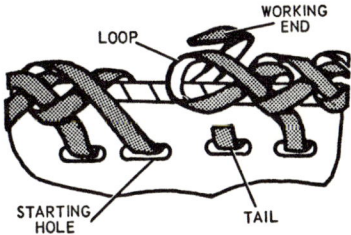

Figure 13-69

Step 4. Bring the working end of the lacing up through the loop, from the back.

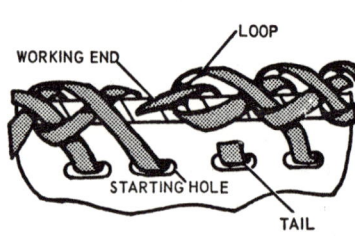

Step 5. Now bring this working end under the cross, or X.

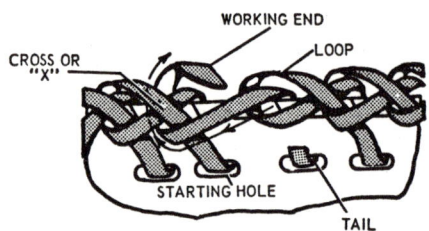

Step 6. Now cross the working end over itself and then down through the loop toward the front.

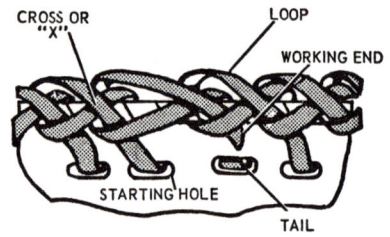

Step 7. Pull the tail out of the hole in the top layer of leather and down between the layers.

Step 8. Put the working end through the hole in the top layer of leather and down between the layers.

Step 9. Adjust this ending stitch to look like the others. Cut the ends, leaving about ½ inch and tuck or glue them to the sides of the leather.

Remember! To end double cordovan, put the lacing through the hole, up through the loop, under the X or cross, and down through loop toward the front and through the hole. Slip the ends between the layers of leather.

BATIK AND TIE DYEING

Therapeutic Implications

Batik and tie dyeing have great appeal for those with limited physical capacity. This art form is particularly useful in a group, where the different skills needed can be found among different members.

Both techniques involve the preparation and use of fabric, the use of color, spatial planning, squeezing out, and dipping.

Minimum physical strength is required, except for the squeezing-out process and the cutting of fabric pieces; therefore, it is appropriate for those with limited physical endurance or generalized physical weakness.

Batiking is more involved than tie dyeing, presenting more of a mental challenge and more opportunity for creativity. It is not the ideal activity for muscle strengthening, because it requires nothing more taxing than brushing on wax, using a light grasp on the brush. The following physical requirements should be noted:

- Cutting of fabric calls for active opening and closing of the hand (a short-term exercise good for improving joint mobility in the hand).

- Tracing a design or drawing it on material requires eye-hand coordination and light grasping of the pencil or stylus.

- Dipping requires minimal strength and joint motion, primarily at the shoulder.

- Appropriate placement of the wax calls for some visual perception to differentiate foreground from background.

- The use of hot wax limits this craft to those who have intact sensation and good judgment about safety.

- Squeezing out the water requires moderate grasp strength of at least one hand, and can encourage elbow pronation and supination when done with two hands.

The cognitive ability required by this craft is fairly simple; the steps of the process can be broken down to simplify learning. For those who cannot readily trace a design, doing a free-form design can be more rewarding because of the interesting effects produced. Reapplication of wax for the second color can be eliminated for those who cannot grasp the reversal process. For someone who benefits from intellectual stimulation, the instruction can be extended to include the chemistry of the dyeing process.

Tie dyeing provides less opportunity for creativity, but is more easily done by a mildly confused person. The cutting requires active use of the hand in opening and closing the scissors. The primary ability required is the bunching and securing of the fabric, which is also a good bilateral activity. Manipulating clothespins is especially useful for increasing grasping and holding strength. The dipping process takes light shoulder motion.

This craft is less adaptable for a person with the use of only one hand, but can be done effectively by two working together.

A visually limited person would find this craft difficult and unrewarding, because there is little or no tactile feedback. Those who have functional use of the hands but lack strength in shoulder and elbow muscles can do the bunching at lap level.

This medium has the advantage of providing pleasure very quickly with a minimum investment of time and effort.

A Batik Scarf

Batik is an ancient textile design technique using a wax resist and dyes to create a pattern on fabric.

Materials

1. electric skillet (or saucepan) with water
2. heavy-duty extension cord
3. metal container for wax
4. flat brushes of various widths
5. basins or large-mouth jars for each color of dye
6. electric iron
7. long-handled spoon for stirring dye baths
8. newspapers or other absorbent paper
9. waxed paper

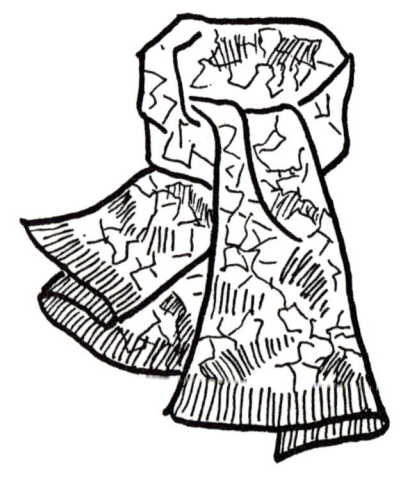

10. dry-cleaning fluid
11. disposable gloves for use with dyes
12. fabric, 12" × 45"
13. thermometer for testing wax temperature
14. wax
15. dyes

Fabric. Silk, linen, wool, cotton, or unbleached muslin can be used (old sheets work well), but no synthetics. The best substitute for silk is 100 % cotton batiste.

Wax. A blend of paraffin (60%) and beeswax (40%) is best. If more crackle is desired, the percentage of paraffin should be increased. Old candles are all right if they are not too deeply colored.

Dyes. Dylon, Batikit or other specialized dyes, or regular fabric dyes such as Putnam, Tintex, and Rit, can be used. (They must be cold-water dyes.)

Procedure

Mix the dyes according to the package instructions.
Heat the wax to 250°F. in the water bath. (The wax is placed in the metal container in the water bath.)
Place the fabric, cut to size, on the waxed paper, which will protect the working surface from hot wax.
Plan the design to be used and either draw it on the fabric with a pencil or place the pattern under the waxed paper, visible through the fabric. Free-form designs, requiring no pattern, can be very effective for beginning projects.
Apply wax to the parts of the pattern that are to remain white, and immerse the fabric in the first dye bath, which should be the lightest color in the planned design.
Leave the fabric in the dye bath until the desired intensity of color is reached. The time will vary with the type of dye used. Remember that colors always appear darker when wet.
Remove the fabric from the dye bath and rinse it under cold water until color no longer appears in the water. Try to avoid removing wax during rinsing.
Allow the fabric to dry before applying the next coat of wax. Drying can be speeded up by use of a hair dryer or any other source of heat if care is taken not to melt the wax.

When the fabric is dry, place it on the waxed paper again and apply wax to the parts that are to remain the color of the first dye bath. Immerse the fabric in the next dye bath.

Repeat this procedure until all the desired colors have been included. The original plan for the design determines how many dye baths and waxings are needed.

The final step usually consists of coating the entire design with wax, crumpling it enough to achieve the amount of crackle desired, and dipping it into a dark dye bath, usually black. Navy blue, dark brown, or dark red could be used, depending on the color scheme.

When the fabric has been rinsed and dried after the final dye bath, the wax must be removed.

Wax Removal. Rub the material between the hands to break off most of the surface wax. Save it for use in future projects. Place the fabric between several layers of newspaper, and iron with a medium-hot iron to melt the remaining wax. Change the paper whenever it becomes saturated with melted wax. Be careful not to place the fabric next to colored ink or extremely dark copy in the paper, because these inks may bleed into the batik design.

Most of the wax can be removed with the hot iron, but if the fabric remains stiff after repeated ironing, use dry-cleaning fluid to remove the remainder.

Scarves should be finished with narrow, rolled hems for soft fabrics, or machine stitching or turning under and blind stitching for heavier materials.

Variations

The fabric can be put in a frame or tacked on a board for wall display when the project is completed.

Larger pieces can be dyed for clothing, but are usually too expensive for group projects.

Adaptations

For those using only one hand, a hem can be ironed in and the work can be put in a clamped embroidery hoop. The fabric can be taped or held in a clipboard to eliminate slippage when applying wax. A free-form design can be used by those with mild coordination problems. Consider the use of only one color dye (the crackling process will create a pleasing effect).

The fabric can be precut by staff members.

Note: Participants with sensory deficits should be closely supervised with this craft.

A Tie-Dyed Place Mat

Materials

1. batiking dye (cold-water dye)
2. 100% cotton fabric
3. large, wide-mouth fruit jar
4. tongs
5. rubber gloves or surgical throw-away gloves
6. clothespins, paper clips, or rubber bands
7. scissors

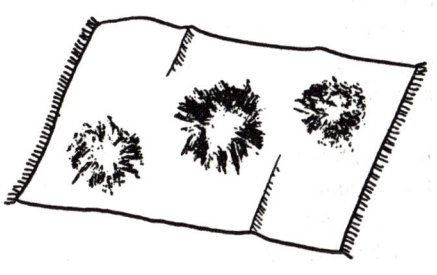

Procedure

Cut the fabric to the desired size for project—a scarf, handkerchief, or place mat.

Mix the dye according to the package instructions and put it in the jar.

Bunch the fabric and fasten the bunches together with rubber bands, clothes pins, or paper clips.

Place Mat Bunched and tied

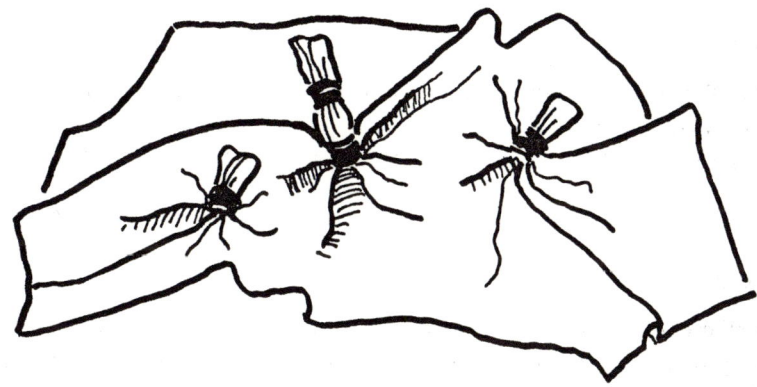

Using the tongs, immerse the fabric in the dye until the desired shade is obtained. (It will be lighter after it dries, so make it darker than desired.) See the directions on the dye package for the required dyeing time.

With the clips or bands still in place, rinse the fabric in cold water until the rinse water is entirely clear.

Squeeze out the fabric and place it in the fixative that comes with the dye. Stir, wait the prescribed time, then rinse with running water until the water is clear.

Squeeze out the water and hang the fabric up to dry with the clips or bands still in place.

Remove the clips or bands after the fabric is dry, then press and hem it.

Variations

More than one color can be used, but this requires planning ahead on how the colors can be placed for the second and third dippings.

A large piece of fabric can be used to create a pleasing design for framing and hanging.

Adaptations

Some people may need assistance in bunching and tying after the places for the design are chosen. Long-handled tongs can be used for dipping and fixing.

An embroidery hoop, stabilized, or a one-hand embroidery frame (see Appendix B) can be used to hold the fabric for hemming after the raw edge has been folded and pressed.

This can be a group project. A one-handed person can bunch the material and hold it while another one slips a clip or clothespin over the gathered fabric.

This is a project that can be done outdoors.

Craft Projects 169

DECORATIVE CONTAINERS

Therapeutic Implications

The activities described in this section vary in their potential for therapeutic use. They are all short-term projects, providing rapid satisfaction and possibly building confidence in residual abilities. For the most part, they are activities requiring more coordination than strength, making them good choices for those with limited muscle power in the upper extremities or with limited endurance.

These crafts are essentially simple tasks that can be learned readily by most people who see them demonstrated. With the exception of the bottle-dipping project, all are structured crafts that require the ability to follow a sequence of steps involving verbal, tactile, or visual demonstrations.

All these projects can be used effectively for a group, but offer little opportunity for individual initiative. They differ somewhat in the kinds of ability required, as follows:

Bottle Dipping

- is easily done with one hand
- requires good coordination for twisting the bottle and dripping the paint
- is too involved to set up for one person's project
- requires fair vision to achieve satisfactory results.

Twine Wrapping

- requires grasping ability in at least one hand to hold the twine and do the gluing
- can be done with primary hand motion if the elbows are supported on the table
- encourages two-hand interaction if wrapping is done half way with one hand and then the task is shifted to the other hand
- encourages greater elbow range if wider pots are used, and encourages greater shoulder range if tall pots are used
- encourages rotary motion at the wrist, through the winding process
- provides tactile feedback because the twine offers a good contrasting texture to the pot, and serves as a guide for those with visual limitations.

Patchwork

- This is excellent for those who need strengthening in grasp and release of the hand. The scissors and fabric provide resistance to both closing and opening of the hand.
- For the one-handed person, the fabric must be stabilized for cutting. Because the patchwork pieces should be small, cutting is generally difficult. Two one-handed persons can work together or the pieces can be precut.
- Brushing on finish is a good gross activity for those who have little control of hand and arm movements.
- Exacting hand control is not required for the placement of the swatches, so this project is good for the visually limited and those with mild coordination problems.

Masking Tape

- This work requires some grasping strength for tearing tape, or the ability to use scissors. It encourages minimal strengthening through the opening and closing of the hand.
- The buffing process encourages the use of elbow flexion and extension.
- Because the tape pieces vary in size and overlap, a person with mild coordination problems can complete the project successfully.
- As tape is fairly flat, a visually impaired person must have a fairly good sense of touch.

Paper Weight

- Minimal strength is required to push decorative items into the clay.
- Some imagination is required for designing and arranging.
- A degree of visual and perceptual ability is needed to judge the size of the arrangement in comparison with the bottle.
- One-handed but well-coordinated people should be able to do this work using paint on the lid for contrast, instead of taping.

Wishing Well

- Hand strengthening can be stimulated by having the participant separate the clothespins.

- Light grasping is required, with potential for improvement in elbow and shoulder range if the pins and bottle are placed higher or farther away on the table.
- The need for exact placement encourages the development of increased dexterity.
- Making the top of the well requires fine dexterity, so those with poor control may need assistance in completing it.

Shell Container

- A participant must be able to make prehensile movements with a fair amount of control to place the shells.
- This project can be used for tactile orientation for the visually impaired by having the participant sort shells according to texture and size before beginning.
- The project can be arranged to improve perception by having the participant alternate the size of the shells as they are applied, work left to right, or work top to bottom.
- A plastic pot can be used for the person with severe visual impairment, so the pot will not have to be painted.

Bottle Dipping

Materials

1. bucket to hold water
2. popsicle or craft sticks
3. waxed paper
4. paper towels and rags for cleanup
5. turpentine
6. oil-base paint, assorted colors including white
7. bottles, clear or in color*
8. florist's clay (can be reused)

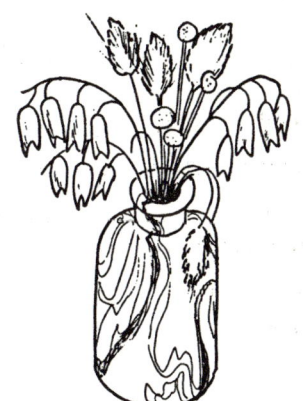

---

*Clear bottles must be painted white and allowed to dry before being dipped in the colors.

Procedure

Fill the bucket with water 2″ or 3″ deeper than the bottle to be dipped.

Dip a stick into the paint and drip it in swirls on the surface of the water. Repeat this with as many colors as desired, or start with two or three colors if the process is unfamiliar.

Fill the mouth of the bottle with florist's clay. Insert one of the popsicle or craft sticks into the clay and be sure that it is stable enough for handling the bottle during dipping.

Dip the bottle into the paint-covered surface of the water twisting it as you raise it. The bottle must be submerged completely, so the neck edge is covered. If the bottle has been painted white first, some interesting effects can be had by just partially dipping the bottle so that some of the white shows, perhaps a quarter or a third above the colors. Or, the white bottle can be dipped at an angle to create another effect.

Place the dipped bottles on waxed paper, leaving the sticks in place until the paint has thoroughly dried. Reuse the clay and sticks.

To change the paint colors: With a paper towel, skim the paint from the surface of the water until it is clear and clean, then continue with new colors.

When finished, fill the bottles with straw flowers or other dried materials.

Adaptations

Once the bottles or cans of paint are opened, this project can easily be done by a one-handed person.

Shell Container

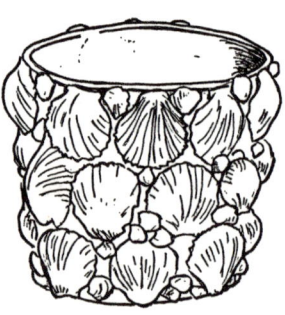

Materials

1. shells, assorted shapes and sizes
2. clay flower pots or plastic pots
3. enamel (white or color)
4. paintbrush
5. white glue

Procedure

Paint the flower pot and allow it to dry thoroughly. (White containers need not be painted.) Glue shells on the outside of the pot with white glue, making attractive designs. Leave the base of the pot free of shells so it can be used either standing or hanging.

Variations

Other containers can be used—plastic drinking glasses (which need not be painted) or regular glasses or jars with attractive shapes.

Scraps of colored glass, bits of wood, and beads or seeds can be used for decorating.

Twine-Wrap Container

Figure 13-70 Starting the Twine

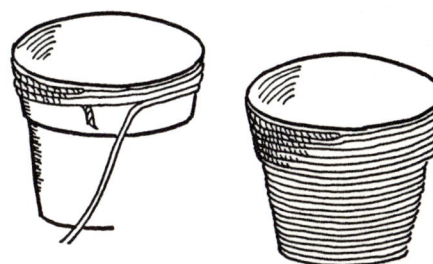

Materials

1. container
2. twine (seine, cable, or sisal)
3. white glue
4. clear acrylic spray

Procedure

Apply the glue with the brush on small areas of the container at a time and wind the twine around the container, starting at the top. Leave the drainage hole uncovered. Spray the finished container with clear acrylic after the glue has dried.

Patchwork Container

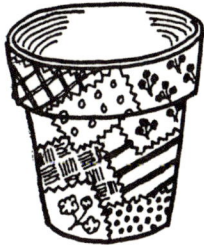

Materials

1. container
2. small swatches of plain or printed material
3. scissors
4. white glue
5. clear acrylic spray

Procedure

Cut the swatches of material to the desired sizes. Apply glue to small areas of the container at a time. Place the swatches in a patchwork design, overlapping if necessary to avoid leaving spaces between patches.

When the glue is thoroughly dry, spray the container with clear acrylic or use a diluted mixture of white glue and water applied lightly with a brush.

Variation

To make a cachepot from a decorated flower pot, close up drainage hole, pour about ¼" of plaster of Paris in pot bottom to secure plug. Let plaster and porous pot dry thoroughly.

Waterproof inside of porous pot by applying 2 or 3 coats of liquid self-polishing floor wax.

Masking Tape Container ("Looks-like-leather" technique)

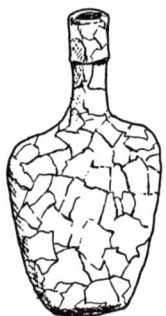

Materials

1. bottle or other container with pleasing shape
2. tan masking tape
3. shoe polish, brown or cordovan

Procedure

Tear tan masking tape in ½" or ¾" pieces and apply over the entire container surface, overlapping edges to give a layered look. Apply several coats of shoe polish, buffing between each coat. The finished container will have the appearance of leather.

An attractive lamp base can be made this way.

Adaptations

Containers can be held, while decorative pieces are being glued in place, by weights such as heavy stones placed in the bottom.

Participants should let the glue get tacky before gluing on the decorative pieces to avoid slippage toward the bottom of the container or off at an angle.

Two one-handed persons can wind the twine, one person turning the container as the other presses the twine into place.

Some assistance might be needed for tearing the masking tape. This can be solved by putting the tape in a heavy dispenser, which will stabilize it so one person can control the tearing.

Paperweight

Materials

1. jars with tightly fitting tops
2. florist's clay
3. plastic flowers and leaves, of a size to fit into the jar
4. marbles
5. seashells
6. chrome tape 2'' wide (or paint) to finish the jar top
7. scissors
8. paper towels to keep hands and work space clean
9. waxed paper or oilcloth to cover working surface

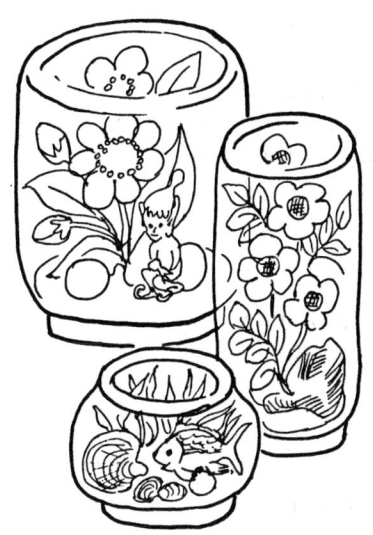

Procedure

Cover the working surface with waxed paper. Fill the jar with water and set it aside. Press the florist's clay firmly into the jar top to form the base for the arrangement. Insert some marbles to add weight, then arrange the flowers, seashells, and perhaps a small figurine, pressing each piece firmly into the clay. Remember that the arrangement will be turned over, so everything must be secure. Look at the completed work from all sides until you are finally pleased with it.

Invert the jar top (with the arrangement), carefully put it on the water-filled jar, and screw it on firmly. Turn the jar upside down.

To finish the paperweight, cover the jar lid with chrome tape or paint it to blend with the arrangement.

Variation

This can be done with a dried arrangement in exactly the same way, but omit the water. Add stones or other heavy material to the arrangement to provide a solid base.

Adaptations

Anchor the jar lid to the working surface with florist's clay. Assist the participant in screwing on the jar lid and applying the chrome tape, or suggest that the lid be painted as the final step, instead of using the tape.

Wishing Well

Materials

1. baby-food jar, small size
2. clip-type clothespins, separated by twisting the halves apart
3. dried flowers or other dried materials
4. narrow ribbon for bow (optional)
5. white glue
6. maple or walnut stain
7. electrical tape (black or red)
8. paintbrushes

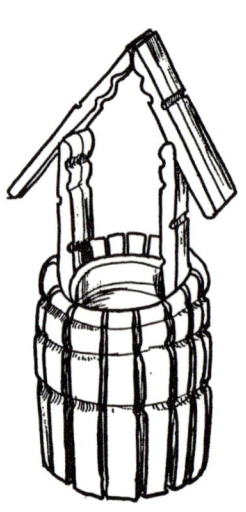

Procedure

Glue the clothespin halves to the outside of the jar, groove sides out. Space them so that there are no large gaps. (See Figure 13-71.)

Clothespin half.

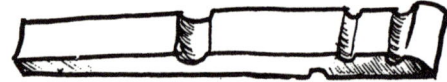

Figure 13-71 Glue half clothespins around baby-food jar.

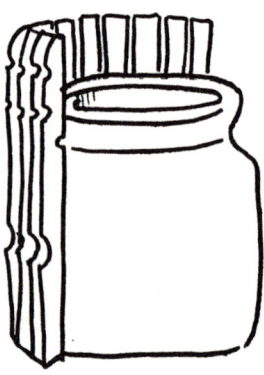

Glue two clothespin halves side by side to make each roof support. Then glue the supports against the sides of the jar, wedging them into the space between the glass and the pins already glued around it. Glue two halves together to form the roof sides; then glue those into an A shape. (See Figure 13-72.)

Two halves glued together.

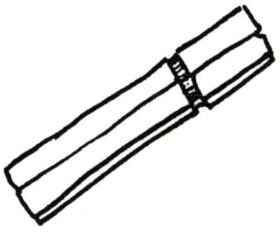

Make use of the grooves wherever possible for firmer adhesion. Allow all glued parts to dry well.

Stain the finished well all over. Apply the tape around the grooves and tie a bow in the side.

The wishing well container can be used for dried arrangements, or filled with water for small plants or flowers. (See Figure 13-73.)

Figure 13-72 Form A-shaped roof and attach to roof supports.

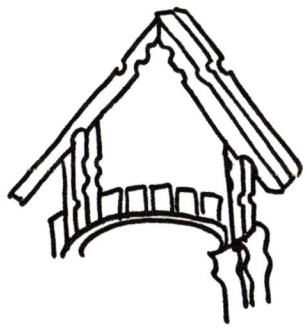

Note: Four halves can be used on each side if a wider roof is desired.

Figure 13-73 Completed Wishing Well

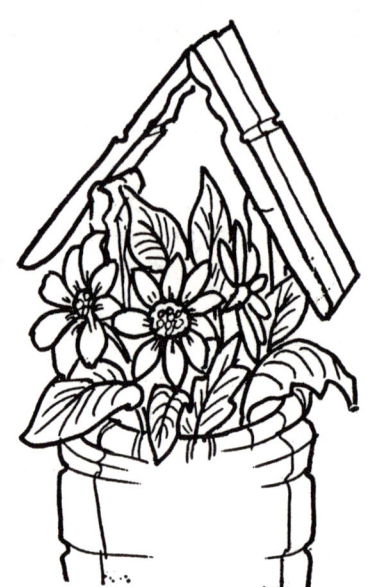

Adaptations

The jar can be anchored on its side with a C-clamp or fixed to the table top with florist's clay. Glue is easier for one-handed people to apply if it is poured into small jars and brushed on. Allow it to get tacky to avoid slippage of the clothespin halves on the rounded surface.

ART

Therapeutic Implications

An art program's greatest value is in providing opportunities for the free expression of feelings and ideas. Proper introduction of the subject and the absence of pressure or implications as to the end product desired can establish the emotional climate needed for such expression.

Painting can be an outlet for frustrations because it gives each person the choice of various sized brushes and large paper; unrestricting techniques, such as spackle painting and loose strokes; and materials, such as paint in contrast to pencil or pen and ink. These mediums can be useful also for participants who lack fine control of the upper extremities and for those who have little artistic ability but are adventurous in experimenting.

The confused participant may require more structure than a typical watercolor or oil painting class might allow. The technique of using masking tape to limit areas of color may be useful for people with this problem.

For those limited in speech, art opens the way to communicate needs and to share a group experience using other senses.

Because drawing and painting provide minimal resistance, they offer little potential for improving physical function, but they do allow the participation of those who are limited in endurance.

Handling a brush, pencil, or pen requires some degree of coordination. Those with weakness in the shoulder and elbow muscles can use a table or lapboard for support.

The visually impaired person would find most painting techniques unrewarding, because there is little tactile feedback. The collage method, however, can provide an opportunity for improving the sense of touch.

Art Activities

Figure 13-74 Art Materials

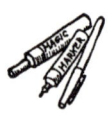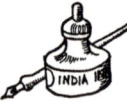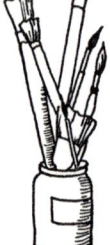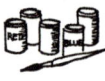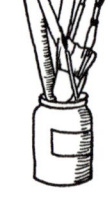

Materials

1. water paints or tempera paints
2. paintbrushes
3. magic markers
4. paper
5. water
6. colored construction paper
7. pen and ink
8. masking tape
9. collage materials: string, bits of cloth, paper clips, rubber bands, tissue paper, etc.
10. scratch-art materials (see Appendix C)

Procedure

The goal is to paint for the joy of it. By following some simple lessons, step by step, beginners can learn to produce satisfying works.

The first step is to stimulate ideas. One way is to paint after listening to music or inspirational words to set a mood for creativity. Participants can examine a person's collection, photographs, prints, flowers from the garden, or even fruits and vegetables, in order to start a discussion that points up differences in form, color, and textures.

Introduce a variety of visual experiments to induce involvement, such as different colored bottles in front of a window or light. Present a variety of sizes and shapes in colored construction paper to be arranged on a black or white background. Immediate decisions and changes are simple, and effective compositions can help overcome timidity or passive viewing.

Introduce paint, brushes, and motion. Spontaneity is important. Work with simple mediums for a start (pen or brush with ink may be a good introduction). Practice bold, accidental strokes, thick and thin, over the entire page. Suggest using the entire page from the beginning, rather than a piecemeal drawing in one corner, then another.

Try the Paul Klee* project called "Take a walk with a line." Start anywhere on the page and move back and forth, in and out, over the whole surface, returning to

---

*Swiss modernist painter and etcher (1879 - 1940).

the starting point to create an artistic doodle. The resulting shapes should be made into a balanced composition with the addition of color in the resulting spaces. Color can be applied with magic markers or tempera.

Experiment in color composition, as a starter. Fold a wet painting of a variety of dripped or splashed tempera colors. Try fold-overs in any direction—vertical, diagonal, or horizontal—quickly before the paint dries. The blend of color and shapes can free the imagination for additions in line for interesting mixed-media results. This can be a good lesson in symmetrical color and design.

Color composition can be the theme for an easy project. In a basic form of abstract art, create a design of various-size boxes or rectangles by arranging three widths of masking tape in a composition of horizontals and verticals. Use strong colors, painted flat or marbleized, covering the entire surface. When the paint is thoroughly dry, strip the tape from the paper. The result is a bold statement in stripes and rectangles.

Visual awareness and perception can be sharpened by suggestions in the ways we look back and forth from the world of nature to the world of art. Simple exercises to encourage awareness of contrasts can be another springboard into ideas. These contrasts can be light and dark, cold and hot, straight and curved, short and tall, or smooth and rough. Associations can do this, too, when used with color: red (roses, sunsets, or fire), yellow (sunlight or flowers), blue (sky, water, "blue" mood), etc.

Paint after a discussion of new viewpoints, such as looking down from high places or looking at the world as an insect would. Create dimension by painting the background and distant things first and close-up things last. Further exploration in paint can be achieved with cardboard cutouts or stencils and with sponge, palette knife, or roller painting.

Scratch Art (see Appendix C) is a good medium for those having little artistic skill. Using pictures from greeting cards or magazines, the participants can scratch out a simple design with a wooden stylus on a sheet of paper that has a black coating. The color beneath the black surface emerges as a picture that has been scratched or etched onto the sheet.

Small pictures can be mounted on cards for stationery, or on construction paper for display. Red, yellow, blue, green, pink and white are suitable colors for Scratch Art work.

Another interesting experiment in painting is the collage, which might be called "layer painting." This method challenges the artist with a variety of surface materials instead of the single paint surface. Overlapping planes and shapes are added to the original foundation with, for example, fabric, newspaper, and photographs. The addition of paint, as the collage progresses, produces the combinations of textures and colors that form a collage painting.

Adaptations

Paper can be taped to the table or stabilized in a clipboard for a one-handed or mildly uncoordinated person.

Tools can be built up with foam rubber, tape, or wooden dowels for those with prehensile or grasp weakness.

A utility holder can be used by those lacking the use of a hand. (See Appendix B.)

Tuning in the participant to utilization of the senses of touch (feeling the form of the object), smell (smelling a flower to be drawn), and vision (bright, bold colors in contrast to cool ones or grays) can stimulate appreciation of line, color, and form.

MOSAICS

Therapeutic Implications

The art of mosaics offers a medium for utilizing fine hand skills and encouraging increased perceptual awareness.

Materials for the mosaic can be chosen to meet the therapeutic goal. For a person capable of only light grasping or limited in dexterity, large tiles or wood pieces may be indicated. For a person who needs to increase fine prehensile skills, smaller mosaic pieces, such as small tiles or seeds, should be selected. (See *Bean Mosaic Kitchen Canister,* following.)

Participants can be asked to cut the materials to be used if resistive motions are needed. This can be done with ceramic-tile cutting, twine cutting for the bean mosaic canister, and sawing wood pieces for wood relief projects.

Tile cutting requires good strength for both opening and closing the hand. Twine cutting can be done with less strength, but can be highly resistive, depending on the weight of the twine. Sawing wood involves all gross muscle groups from the shoulder to the hand, and is highly resistive.

Designs for the mosaics can be selected to meet individual needs or abilities. A simple alternating color pattern (checkerboard type, as in Figure 13-75) or an alternating-line design (one row black, one row white) can be used for those who are more limited.

Figure 13-75 Checkerboard Design

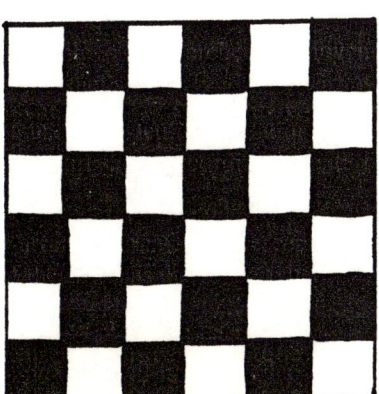

More complicated designs and less structure, using different materials or varying the tile or bean and seed shapes, can be used for the less confused or for the more creative participant. (See Figure 13-76.)

The use of visual perception can be encouraged through this art form. Sorting materials by texture, color, and size is a useful exercise in preparation for the project. Lining up the materials in the selected space requires judgment in spatial relationships as well as verticality and depth awareness.

The visually impaired can gain increased tactile awareness by using materials with various textures.

A project can be selected of the proper complexity to enhance concentration and memory. Those limited in speech can learn the technique with visual demonstration and examples.

Mosaics involve designing and placing varied materials on a base. Interesting results can be achieved with beans, peas, stones and pebbles, wood, tiles, glass, beads, paper, and grasses. A simple design can be made on any kind of hardboard or Masonite. Boxes, bookends, trivets, and other commercially available bases can be purchased for the mosaic application. A coat of glue is brushed on and color and texture are added with various materials. The surrounding area should contrast with the composition.

The bean mosaic work is particularly good for sorting, matching, and tactile discrimination, and is useful for those who have perceptual deficits or for those limited in vision who need to increase their touch discrimination.

Figure 13-76 Complex Design

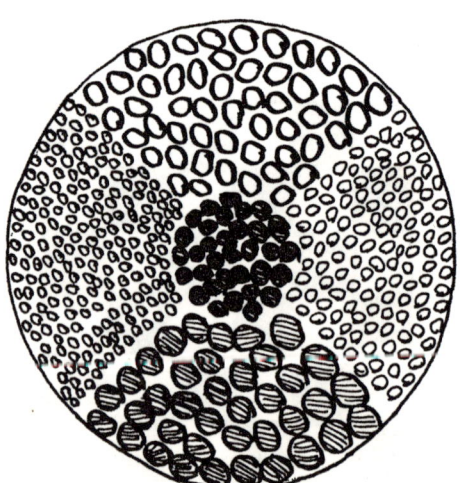

For a wood relief, it is possible to use scraps of wood that require only sanding and finishing. The sanding process can improve strengthening of muscles and increase range of motion, depending on the placement of the pieces.

Hand sawing requires a great deal of strength, so the possibilities are limited for those with more than slight strength loss. For a person with a central nervous system dysfunction, such as a stroke, a staff member must always observe what is happening with the affected side when the participant is doing a forceful activity with the unaffected side. Exertion may induce more spasticity on the affected side. If this activity is used for gross grasp and release placement, it is necessary to make sure the participant can release the block as well as pick it up. If there is tight grasp without release, it is more beneficial to use extension (pushing away) instead of pulling motions.

Bean Mosaic Kitchen Canister

Materials

1. metal canister 7″ high, 6″ diameter
2. twine, natural color
3. white glue
4. glue brush
5. popcorn, mung beans, kidney beans, yellow split peas, soybeans, etc.
6. enamel, reddish-brown, small bottle
7. spray varnish
8. black waterproof marker

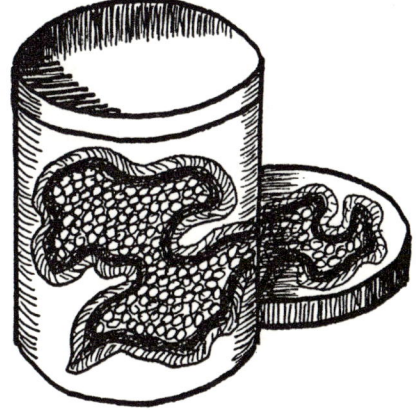

Procedure

Draw an abstract swirl design directly on the canister. Leave ½″ at the top plain.

Cut the twine into varying lengths and soak it in a solution of three parts glue to one part water for several minutes. Apply the twine on top of the inked swirl design to outline the work area. Brush glue onto the outlined area and allow it to become tacky. Allow to dry. Apply the beans and other assorted dried material within the twine design, varying the colors and shapes to fit into the design. More detail can be added by repeating the process of applying the soaked twine and continuing with the addition of the dried material.

When the glue is completely dry, paint the remaining areas of the canister with enamel or fill in the plain spots with random swirls of soaked twine.

When the paint and glue are completely dry, add a final finish of two or three coats of spray varnish.

Decorate the cover to match the work done on the canister.

Variations

Boxes, bottles, and plaques can be decorated in the same manner.

Adaptations

Use the larger beans and seeds for easier handling by those with limitations.

Those who use only the left hand should be provided with left-handed scissors. (See Appendix B.)

Pre-gluing the twine will assist the visually limited, as will the selection of distinct colors and sizes of beans. One type of bean or seed and one space can be done at a time if limitations of vision cause confusion.

The container can be weighted down by placing stones in it. If the top is put on it and it is placed sideways, the stones will stabilize it. Or, the canister could be clamped to the table on a cushioned surface.

Shorter, more manageable lengths of twine can be used, or the area not seeded can be painted instead of being filled in with twine.

Brush-on varnish can be used instead of spray varnish if ventilation is inadequate.

Note: This is a poor activity for those having more than minor coordination problems.

Tile Hot Plate

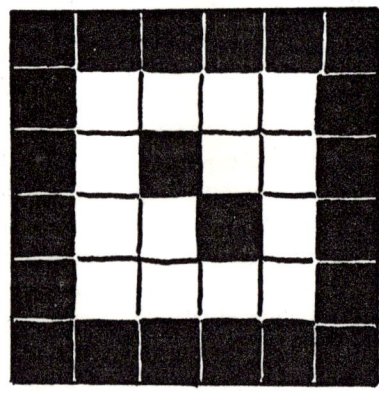

Materials

1. wood or Masonite base, 6″ × 6″
2. grout
3. white glue
4. tile cutter
5. tiles, assorted colors
6. water to mix with grout
7. tongue depressors
8. damp sponge
9. grout sealer

Procedure

A design can be drawn and transferred onto the base, or the arrangement can be decided as the pieces are set.

Dip or brush glue on each piece and set the pieces one at a time. Allow space (1/16'' to 1/8'') between tiles for grouting. Let the glue dry thoroughly.

Mix the grout with water to the consistency of heavy cream and apply it over the entire tiled surface. (The grout can be colored with food coloring or acrylic paints.) Use tongue depressors or a flat tool to scrape off the excess grout, keeping the tool flat on the tops of the tiles. Let it dry.

With a damp sponge, do the final cleaning of the tiled surface. Apply the grout sealer with a brush, or spray it on.

Adaptations

- Large tiles can be used for those who lack fine prehension.
- Tiles can be placed on a foam surface (old foam-backed placemats are useful) to facilitate picking them up.
- For visually or perceptually impaired people, colors should be chosen with sharp contrast, such as white and black.
- The space to be glued can be marked off with tongue depressors, masking tape, or heavy black lines to provide a guide for confused or visually impaired participants.

Wood Relief

Materials

1. saw for cutting wood base
2. wood or Masonite for base
3. discarded pieces of wood or junk (bottle caps, corks, thread spools, door knobs, etc.)
4. heavy white glue, such as Sobo
5. flat latex paint or varnish for sealing wood
6. semi-gloss latex paint for base, if desired
7. brushes for glue and finish
8. ½'' half-round doweling or ½'' framing if desired
9. ½'' screw eyes
10. wire for hanging

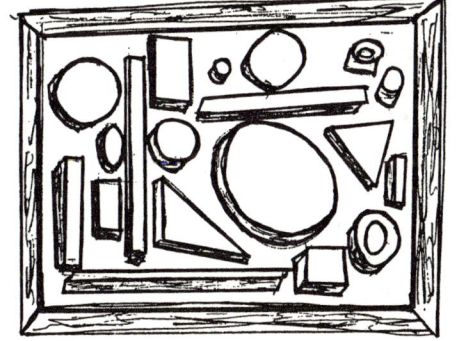

Procedure

1. Measure and cut out the base. The size is optional, but 16″ × 20″ gives a nice area for working.
2. Sand the base until the flat surface and edges are smooth.
3. Paint with flat latex or varnish the top and edges of the wood base to seal the wood. Let it dry thoroughly.
4. Apply semi-gloss paint if a color is desired, or add a second coat of varnish.
5. Lay out assorted pieces of wood or junk on the base, and arrange them as desired.
6. If any of the pieces of wood are to be colored, sand and paint them before gluing. If a natural look is preferred, glue them first and varnish the whole piece later.
7. Brush glue on the pieces to be applied to the base and set them in place.
8. If a frame is desired, cut it out and miter the corners. Finish it (preferably in a color contrasting with the base) and glue and nail it to the base.
9. Attach screw eyes and wire to the back for hanging.

Adaptations

Large pieces of wood can be clamped down for sanding. A large sand block can be clamped to the table for independent sanding of straight pieces by a one-handed or slightly uncoordinated person.

Painting or varnishing can be eliminated and rub-on wax can be applied after the piece is assembled.

Participants can dip pieces in glue if handling of the glue bottle or brush is difficult.

MODELING WITH CLAY, DOUGH, AND CORNSTARCH

Therapeutic Implications

The use of clay and bread dough has proved to be quite successful as therapy for the physically disabled as well as for psychiatric patients.

The approach used in introducing these projects makes considerable difference in the way they are received. Clay and dough modeling may meet resistance at first, particularly from older people who may consider it "messy child's play," with associations from their elementary school days, and (except for people with an art background) from those who usually prefer doing something useful.

There are people who refuse to be involved with this medium, and it is important to accept this, because freedom of choice and the opportunity to make decisions is therapeutic in itself.

Experience in using this medium has demonstrated that it is usually received better in a group in which all the members are participating. Another factor in the use of this craft is how often people participate. If they come only once a week, short-term projects are essential. If they are paying for their materials and instruction, they will usually be more insistent about expecting usable results.

Having several samples of attractive finished projects on display is often good for motivation. One may begin the class with a film, a display, or a discussion of the usefulness of the product. For the scientific-minded, a discussion of the properties of clay, bodies, and glazes might provide some incentive. The chance to take home a finished project is also a help. Beginning projects can be planned around small objects, such as beads and pendants to be gaily painted and strung, or a small bon-bon dish that can be decorative and useful.

Ceramics work is an excellent resistive activity for exercise of the upper extremities. Positioning of the project is important in encouraging use of shoulder, elbow, and wrist motions (e.g., placing clay on a table rather than in the lap on a lapboard, and farther away rather than close to the body). People who need strengthening for the fine muscles in the hand can benefit by making pinch pots or doing any other modeling. The size and texture of the clay can be adapted for strengthening the hand. Baker's clay (see *Bread Dough Wreath* for the recipe) may be more appropriate for those with less strength.

People with joint limitations in the hand, wrist, or elbows would profit by using the slab method, in which the clay is rolled. (See *Working with Clay*, following.) Full extension (opening) of the fingers and wrist is encouraged by holding the rolling pin in the middle of the clay or dough and rolling towards oneself; pushing the pin away encourages elbow extension.

For a person with poor coordination, one-piece projects that use the slab method may be better. A template (pattern) made of heavy cardboard can be put on a piece of rolled clay to facilitate cutting with a blunt tool. The use of an overglaze on bisque is sometimes advisable, because the glaze can be dabbled on, overlapped, and built up without precision and the result can still be an attractive finish. The piece must be stabilized when glazing, by putting it in a shallow container (like a pie tin) and clamping the container to the table. Most people have better control if they can work close to the body; therefore, a lapboard or elevating tables can be useful. (See Appendix B.) If there is restricted joint motion, positioning the work closer is crucial.

Some people seem to be able to manage only repetitive activities made up of rhythmic or automatic movements, such as rolling or pounding clay, and may require an impetus (such as the instructor's hands on the participant's) to start the movement.

For the person with little hand strength, the finishing process of glazing or painting may be more appropriate than the preliminary work. Some craft supply houses have ceramic figures that have been bisque-fired and are ready for the final stage. Working with these is preferable to using molds to make the ceramic figure, which can be tricky and usually must be done by staff members.

The exercise value of this medium is obvious, but as one deals with the whole person it is important to realize that psychological aspects are equally important. Many disabled people are understandably depressed by their loss of function and have difficulty in adjusting to it. Working with clay can be important as an outlet for expressing and working out the resulting frustration, even though the finished work may not appear useful or attractive. This craft can be a structured one (in which certain steps are followed with a specific end project in mind) or as an unstructured one (in which the participants are allowed to do with the medium what they feel like doing). A participant's work can be a subject for discussion with a staff member or group members, if the participant is amenable. Sometimes it is enough that the person has just been able to participate in the physical activity without trying to describe what it means. As working with feelings and interpreting them can be dangerous, it is generally advisable to let the participant control the discussion, if it takes place.

Wedging clay requires strength and energy, and for angry, frustrated participants it is often a good outlet for venting feelings. Those who are consistently negative or restless often are more in control and relaxed after a warm-up period of preparing clay.

People with speech problems often get positive feedback from working with clay as an unstructured or creative activity. They can be shown the techniques and the tools, and allowed more flexibility and less structure. If such a person is working in a more structured group, the instructor must be prepared to accept the results of the person's work. The staff member may have to help in handling the clay and producing various shapes. The participant's end product should be given some positive response by the staff, and will often be found to be useful. What looks like an oddly shaped blob may be used in a wind chime, or what looks like a container of irregular size can be used for a dried-flower or shell arrangement. The finishing, particularly the glazing, can often change the character of the original piece. It is important that the final decision on the work be made by the participant, however. Although the staff should feel free to make suggestions, the person who produced it may be satisfied with it as it is.

The disabilities within a group often limit the projects that can be undertaken. However, there is a wide range of complexity in ceramics. For those with limited attention span and those with poor self-esteem, short projects must be used. Working with bread dough meets this requirement, whereas clay projects take longer because of the drying and firing.

Smaller projects, such as beads or cookie-cutter cut-outs for mobiles or wind chimes, are better for those with limited concentration and those needing more immediate satisfaction.

An important consideration in using this medium is the comfort of the participant. Those with joint diseases such as arthritis may find that the dampness of the clay increases joint stiffness. If so, baker's clay, which is less damp and less resistive, may be more appropriate. If a participant continues to complain, a different craft should be tried.

Another precaution is that some persons with dry skin or skin diseases may be irritated by certain foreign bodies in the clay, or by its drying quality. The clay can be handled with surgical throw-away gloves, but then the heat of the gloves may cause trouble.

Certain types of clay have more odor than others and some people (e.g., those with multiple sclerosis or cystic fibrosis) can be affected adversely. For all participants, including the staff, good ventilation is important for this activity.

Working with Clay

Materials

1. self-hardening clay
2. modeling tools (nut picks, large nails, toothpicks, orange sticks, etc.)
3. sponges
4. rolling pin, 1" diameter dowel, or section of old broom handle
5. plaster bats* (optional)
6. oilcloth for a working surface, tacked to a board or taped to the table
7. rags and cheesecloth

---

*Made by pouring plaster of Paris at least 1" thick into greased 9" pie tins. Remove when hard and use as a movable base for shaping and drying objects.

8. knife
9. ruler
10. textured cloth, burlap, or other rough material
11. plastic bags or wrap

Procedure

Coil Method. Form a small ball of clay and place it on the oilcloth working surface. With the hand flat and rigid and the fingers held tightly together, roll the lump of clay back and forth into a ½" coil. Cover each finished coil with a damp

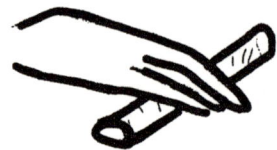

cloth until the desired number has been made. The clay is the right consistency when it rolls smoothly without bumping or jerking, and does not show cracks.

To make a clay pot, form the base from either a spiral of coils or a flat base about ½" thick (rolled out with a rolling pin). Scratch and moisten the base where the first coil is to be applied. (The moistening is omitted for non-hardening clay or Plasticine.) Then wind the coil around the base and weld it. Scratch and moisten as the additional coils are placed on top of one another around the base. Cut the ends of the coils at an angle so they fit together smoothly; then scratch, moisten, and weld.

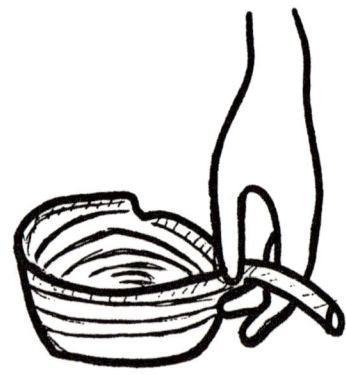

When the desired shape is reached, scrape and sponge the work until it is smooth. When it is in the leather-hard state (moist but firm), the pot can be decorated by incising a design with tools or fingers or by using rolled strings of clay for a relief design.

Pinch-Pot Method. Hold a ball of clay in one hand or place it on a plaster bat. Push the thumb into the center of the ball and turn the ball of clay around and around while pressing the thumb on the inside and the fingers on the outside. The ball will deepen as the walls are built up.

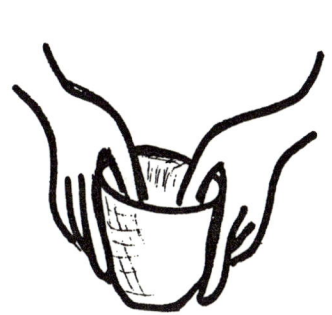
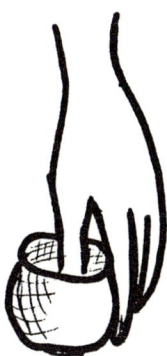

Try to keep the walls of equal thickness so drying will be even. If the bowl has been shaped in the hand, flatten the base by tapping it on a flat surface. The shape can be altered to oval or oblong, or it can be fluted.

Use tools to incise a design when the clay is still moist but firm. Or, add a raised design by scratching the surface and adding pieces.

Slab Method. Place a ball of worked-up clay (kneaded and squeezed in the hands until it is pliable and does not crack) between two pieces of wood of equal thickness on the oilcloth or plaster bat. The required thickness depends on the object to be made. The two pieces of wood space the rolling pin (which rolls on top of them), so they must be just as thick as the desired thickness of the slab. Roll out the clay with a rolling pin to form the slab. For decorative tiles, a candy dish, or a

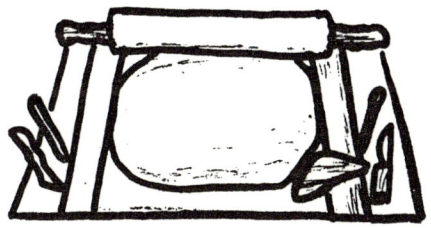

box, the slab should be about ⅜″ thick. For slab animals, tree ornaments, or package tie-ons, it should be ¼″ thick. Slabs ¾″ thick are required for book ends and heavier projects.

Slab Method Using a Clay Hump. Form a clay hump in the shape and size the finished bowl, candy dish, or ash tray is to be. Cover the hump with cheesecloth.

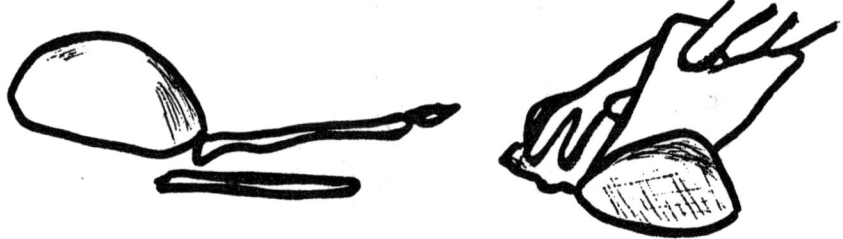

Roll a slab of clay of the desired thickness and drape it over the covered hump. (The cheesecloth prevents the two pieces from sticking together.) Cut away the excess clay at the bottom of the hump and shape it up and around what will be the rim of the bowl.

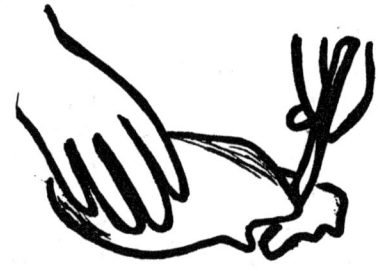

When the clay is firm enough to handle (it will shrink away from the hump), remove it for finishing. Smooth it with a sponge, incise a design, or add pieces for a relief design.

An inverted bowl, greased with Vaseline or Crisco, can be used instead of the cheesecloth-covered clay hump. The clay will shrink away from the bowl when it is ready to be handled for finishing.

To make a hanging pocket for dried arrangements, make a free-form base from clay rolled to a thickness of ⅜" or ¾." The pocket can be made from a ¼" thick slab formed by placing the slab over the clay hump or bowl, as described. Weld the base and pocket together by scratching and moistening the base at the points where the pocket will adhere and applying slight pressure when joining the pieces. The pocket can be decorated while it is over the hump (in the leather-hard state) or after it has been welded to the base.

Make a hole in the top of the base with a large nail before the clay starts to dry.

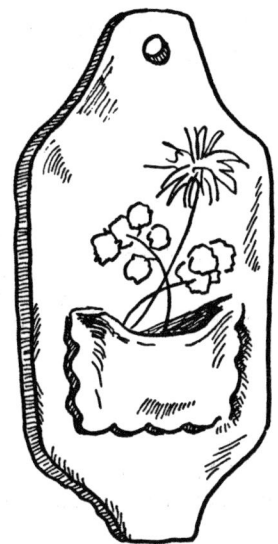

Carefully place some crumpled newspaper in the "pocket," after welding it, to make it more secure during the drying.

To make tree ornaments, package tie-ons, or costume jewelry: Roll the clay to approximately ¼" thickness. Put a cardboard pattern on top of the clay and cut around it, or use cookie cutters. If an ornament is to be hung, pierce a hole at the top for string before the clay starts to dry. Clay shrinks, so be sure the hole is adequate for a string or wire hanger.

To make jewelry, glue jewelry findings (pin backs, clasps, earring clips, etc.) onto the backs of the dried pieces of clay with Duco cement, and the objects can be finished with paint and acrylic spray. Jewelry findings are available in most hobby stores or from craft suppliers.

To make figures, a lump of clay on a plaster bat can be shaped with fingers and tools and coils can be used for some of the parts, which are welded together after scratching and moistening.

Things to remember:

- When clay pieces are joined, they should be of the same dampness; otherwise, they will separate as they dry.
- Unfinished pieces should be kept in plastic bags with a wet sponge between working periods.
- A straight or flat form should be allowed to dry slowly, with a damp cloth or paper towel over it, so it does not warp. (This does not apply to kiln firing.)

Glazing. If a project is to be fired in a kiln, ceramic glazes can be used to give the project a hard, waterproof finish. Specific information on glazing should be obtained from companies that deal in ceramic supplies, because glazes vary and different kilns produce different effects. In general, underglazes are used on greenware (unfired clay), usually where detail is desired. Overglazes are used on bisque (clay that has been fired but not glazed).

If overglaze is used on top of underglaze, it must be transparent so the design will show through.

When using glazes, the work area should be free of dust and the work should be handled as little as possible. (Oil or grease may affect the flow of the glaze in firing, causing air bubbles to form.)

Turntables with heavy bases make glazing easier and reduce handling. These are available at ceramic supply houses, but Rubbermaid turntables or Lazy Susans can be used instead.

Underglaze is generally brushed on (with brushes used for ceramics only). Overglaze may be brushed or dipped. It is important with overglaze to apply several overlapping coats, dappled on in short strokes, making sure there is enough glaze on the brush to cover. In firing, the amount of glaze is reduced, so one must be sure to cover the object well.

The finished color of the glazed product may differ somewhat from the color applied before firing. If possible, glazed samples of each color should be used for comparison.

In some communities, ceramic firing is available for a fee at ceramic supply houses or art instruction centers.

Adaptations

A plaster bat (mentioned previously) can be used as the working surface, eliminating the difficulty of moving the project for a one-handed or uncoordinated person. The bat should be thick enough (1" at least) to give weight and stability. It also provides a good drying surface.

For those participants using only one hand, or with evident weakness, a pizza roller (being light) is easy to handle for rolling the clay. For the uncoordinated participant, a heavy rolling pin is better because it is more stable. (Caution: Any use of tools by a poorly coordinated participant calls for careful monitoring.)

The coil method requires even shaping of coils, and the pinch or slab method is preferred for those participants using only one hand.

For those with visual limitations but with good sensation, clay is a good medium, because it provides tactile feedback.

Templates are helpful if precise forms are desired.

Craft Projects 197

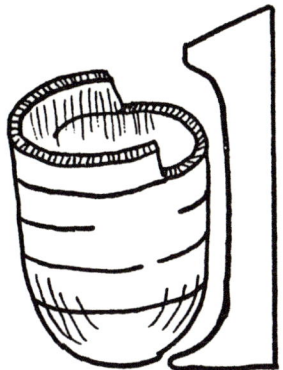

Decorating can be kept simple; ridged shells, paper clips, stamping tools, etc., can be pressed into leather-hard clay to produce interesting textures.

A single color is best for painting or glazing a piece. Textured glazes are preferable for those who are unable to judge color.

Participants should be oriented to tools and materials before a project is initiated. Clay beads are a good beginning project. The use of a stabilized nail for making uniform holes for stringing is described further in this section.

The confused or disoriented participant can benefit from samples. Give one direction at a time, orally, and demonstrate the technique, repeating if necessary.

Bread Dough Animals

Materials

1. paper for patterns
2. tracing paper
3. pencil
4. ruler
5. breadboard
6. rolling pin
7. paintbrushes, one small fine-pointed and one small flat
8. sewing needle
9. narrow velvet ribbon
10. acrylic paints, pink, orange, and green
11. bread dough (for recipe, see *Bread Dough Wreaths*)

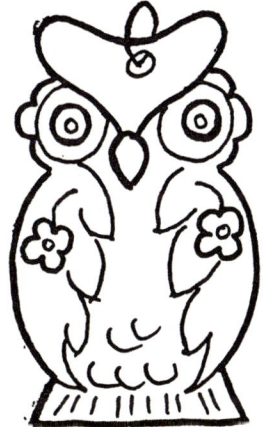

12. aluminum foil
13. plastic wrap
14. small kitchen knife
15. spatula
16. toothpicks
17. cookie sheet
18. potato peeler or any tool with a U-shaped scoop end
19. white glue
20. polyurethane gloss varnish
21. sewing thread
22. thin wire for hangers

Procedure

Enlarge the patterns (Figure 13-76) by copying them onto squared paper, letting each square in the patterns equal a 1″ square for the finished work. The heavier lines indicate outlines and separate dough pieces which will later be placed on the animal shape. The finer lines indicate markings to be made with a toothpick.

Trace the designs onto regular tracing paper and cut them out.

Roll out the dough to ⅜″ thickness on a floured breadboard. Place the pattern tracings lightly on the dough. Mark around the tracings with a toothpick.

Figure 13-76 Patterns for Bread Dough

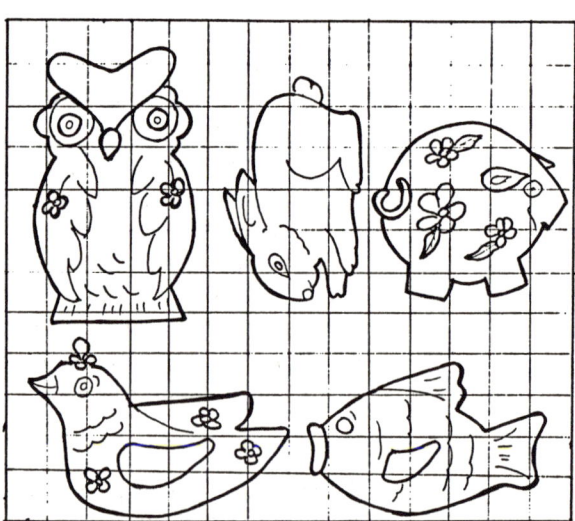

Remove the tracings. Using a knife, cut out the outline of each shape. Place the shapes on a foil-covered cookie sheet with a spatula. With a toothpick, mark all the fine lines, such as for ears and mouths, the owl's body lines, chick's beaks, rabbit's inner ear, etc. Go deep into the dough, but be careful not to go through it.

Use the toothpick to make holes in the eye centers. Narrow coils of dough made by rolling between the hands will do for the owl's eye and pig's tails. Stick all the pieces in place, after moistening the dough at the contact surfaces so they will adhere securely.

Cut pieces of wire 1¼" long. Bend them into loops and put glue on the ends. Insert one into the top of each ornament to serve as a hanger.

Bake the pieces within an hour after making them. If any cannot be baked immediately, cover them with plastic wrap.

Bake the pieces at 300° F. Check after one hour and until done. Cool. Then paint flowers, leaves, eyes, and the other features shown on the illustrations. When they are dry, seal the pieces on all sides and edges with two coats of varnish, allowing them to dry between coats.

Make ribbon hangers.

Variations

Any piece that can be made from a clay-like substance can be made from bread dough: beads, small candy dishes, and so on. Cookie cutters can be used for shapes.

Adaptations

For the person with the use of only one hand, flattened clay can be put on a piece of Styrofoam and toothpicks can be put through the eyes or two other spots, where there could be openings (such as the center of a flower), to stabilize the clay piece for working. A similar technique can be used for the painting and varnishing.

After the shapes have been baked, they can be anchored to the working surface with florist's clay for painting and varnishing.

For the person with visual or perceptual impairments, the fine line pattern may be too difficult. In that case, use a heavy cardboard pattern for the basic shape and narrow lines cut out of the cardboard (like a stencil) to give minimum detail, such as eyes, nose, and wings. The participant can usually be oriented to the openings in the cardboard, through which a dull tool can be pressed. As noted for the clay projects, one-color decorating can be done, or stencils can be used if more detail is desired.

If this is used as a group project, the more limited participants can make the basic shapes and the more functional participants can supply the details.

Bread Dough Wreath

Materials

1. bread dough (see recipe, following)
2. mixing bowl
3. plastic wrap
4. cookie sheet
5. aluminum foil
6. rolling pin
7. toothpicks
8. fork
9. knife
10. wire rack
11. varnish or shellac
12. paint brush, 1"
13. whole cloves
14. epoxy cement

Recipe for Bread Dough

4 cups flour to start. Add more as needed.
1 cup salt
1½ cups warm water
1 heaping teaspoon instant tea or coffee for color

Mix the flour and salt together. Add the tea or coffee to the warm water, dissolve it well, and let it cool. Then add it to the flour mixture, mixing it well and kneading it until it is smooth. Roll the dough into a ball and cover it with plastic wrap to keep it moist.

Procedure

Cover the cookie sheet with aluminum foil. Preheat the oven to 300° F.

Pinch off a large piece of dough, roll it into a long sausage shape, then form it into a circle on the cookie sheet. Wet the ends and press them together. The circle may be any size desired, but save enough dough to make the ornaments. The wreath without decoration is about 8" in diameter, with a 5" diameter center opening, and is about ½" thick.

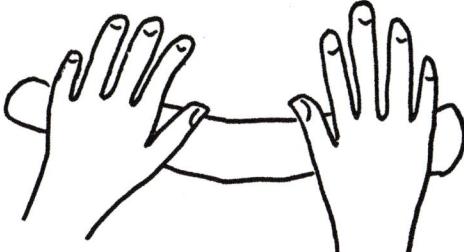

To decorate the wreath, pinch off a piece of dough and roll it out with the rolling pin or flatten it with the hands to about ¼" thickness. Cut out the leaf shapes with a knife and score each leaf with a knife to mark the vein lines. Moisten the back of each leaf with a little water and press it onto the wreath.

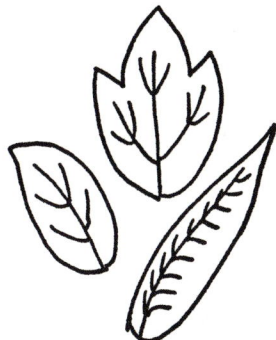

Make the largest fruits next—apples, pears, and peaches. Press whole cloves into the dough for the stems and core ends of the fruit. For stems of apples and pears, push the bud end of the clove into the dough, leaving the stem end out. For the core ends, press in the stem end of the clove, exposing just the bud, from which the ball of the clove has been removed. Wet the wreath circle and attach the fruit pieces. Fill in the spaces with clusters of grapes, strawberries, nuts, and a few plums. Imprint texture and lines with toothpicks or a fork.

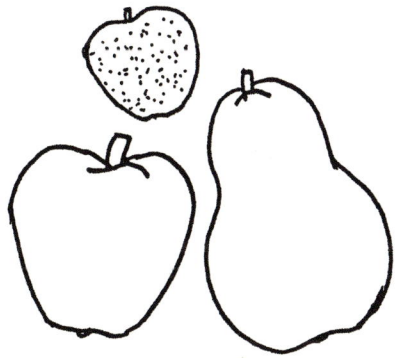

To make the bow, roll out the dough to ¼" thickness. Cut a long strip, about 20"-24" long and 1¼" wide. Fold and pinch the strip into a bow and cut away the ends. Place the bow separately on a foil-covered cookie sheet.

Bake the wreath and bow in a preheated 300° F. oven for three hours or until it is completely dry and hard. If the bow is done before the wreath, tear the foil and remove the bow from the oven.

Place the finished pieces on a wire rack to cool. Peel off the foil. Leave them on the rack for several days in a dry place.

Coat the wreath and bow separately with varnish or shellac. When dry, cement the bow to the wreath with epoxy cement, as directed on package.

Note: Before mixing a large recipe of bread dough, the following can be made up to get the feel of working with dough:

3 slices white bread with crusts removed
3 tablespoons white glue
1 teaspoon glycerine

Crumble the bread and work in the glue and glycerine until the mixture becomes claylike and will hold a shape. Experiment with small leaves and flowers in the palm of the hand or on waxed paper on a flat surface.

By working slowly back and forth, to keep the roll even, a one-handed person can make the sausage shape. Scoring the leaves, inserting the cloves, shaping the smaller pieces needed as fillers, and using the brush for the varnish can also be done by a one-handed person. With patience and practice, the shaping of the larger pieces of fruit can be mastered.

For the visually limited, cardboard patterns can be used on top of the clay as a guide for the shapes; vein lines can be eliminated. If placement of the shapes is a problem, a circle of bread dough can be sectioned off by imprinting shallow lines, or a cardboard stencil can be put over the circle, section by section, as the shapes are added.

This is not a good project for people with poor coordination. For those with limited strength, it is a better medium than clay.

This project is a good one for groups of people assisting one another.

Mexican Jewelry and Dolls

Materials

1. Creative Clay (see recipe, next section)
2. nails or wire
3. acrylic paint, assorted colors
4. shellac

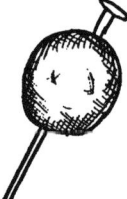

Beads

Mold Creative Clay into shapes for beads, then insert a straightened paper clip, piece of wire, or nail through it to form a hole. Let it remain in the bead until finished. Either allow the beads to dry naturally or pre-heat an oven to 350°, turn it off, and put the clay piece on a rack in the oven. Half an hour in the warm oven should be enough to make the beads dry and hard. Paint them with gay and wild colors, using enamel paint, poster paint, or felt-tip pens. After painting, apply one or two coats of shellac for a professional looking finish. Slip the beads from the wire, and string.

Bracelets

Roll the clay and flatten it out to the thickness desired. Cut it in strips long enough to form a circle that will slip over the hand, and join the ends together after moistening and grooving them with a paper clip. If the bracelet is to be open-ended, allow for slipping the wrist through the opening. Dry as described above.

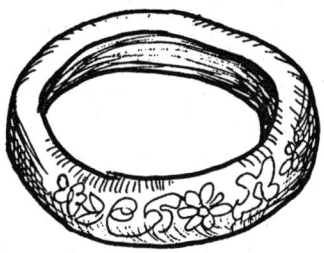

Doll or Puppet Head

Start with a ball or oval of clay. Make the features, and when satisfied with the results, scrape out as much of the inside of the head as possible in order to lighten

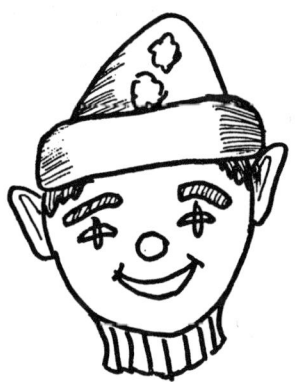

the weight. The neck is added by joining a strip of clay to the base of the head, moistened and grooved as usual. Larger pieces need a longer drying-out period before painting and finishing. Flesh-colored paint should be used for the dolls.

Variations

If the beads are to be strung on thongs or heavy cord, large nails should be used through the centers, instead of paper clips. Pendants can be made by rolling out the clay and making free-form shapes or by using cookie cutters. Make holes for hanging before the pieces are dried.

Adaptations

Adaptive devices to assist the one-handed participant and the visually limited in bead making can be constructed in two ways:
1. Take the lid from a large glass coffee container (at least 10 oz. size) and remove the inside paper disc. With a 4″ common nail (flat-headed), puncture a hole in the center of the disc. Push the nail through the hole and, with the point of the nail up, reinsert the paper disc in the coffee lid. (Use some white glue to fasten the disc firmly to the metal top.) When the glue is dry, make a mixture of plaster of Paris and fill the metal top to the rim, supporting the nail in place if necessary. Let this harden, preferably overnight, and be sure the plaster is dry before using the item. Use florist's clay to anchor the stabilized nail to the table.
2. Stabilize a nail by driving it through the center of a ¾″-1″ thick board. With the point of the nail up, the board can be anchored to the table with a C clamp.

To use either device, roll the clay into a ball, insert it over the point of the nail, shape the bead, then transfer it to a nail of the same size for drying. Remove the dried beads and return them to the plaster-based nail for painting. Greasing the nails before use will keep the clay from sticking.

Some people might have difficulty in making a bracelet, particularly if they are using one hand or if they are visually impaired. They can be assisted in shaping the elongated piece into a circle if they are provided with a plastic detergent bottle (held in a vise) to use as a base to form the bracelet evenly. If the bottle has been greased, the clay will slip easily over the narrowed top for drying.

Stringing the beads may present problems for a one-handed person. If the beads are put into a shallow container or on a soft, thick surface (such as foam), they can be picked up more easily. A method for one-handed knotting is described at the end of the *Stitchery* section.

The plaster-based nail will enable the visually impaired to make beads (of a bulky nature at first). As the process becomes more familiar, smaller sized nails can be set in plaster or the participant may be able to work without this assistance. The beads can be grooved or pinched for texture.

Creative Clay (Cornstarch Recipe)

Materials

1. recipe:
   1 cup cornstarch
   2 cups (1 lb.) baking soda
   1½ cups cold water
2. saucepan
3. spoon for stirring
4. plate for cooling clay
5. damp cloth
6. measuring cup
7. rolling pin (optional)
8. knife or cookie cutter
9. paints (acrylics, water colors, or poster paints) or felt-tip pens
10. clear nail polish, varnish, or shellac

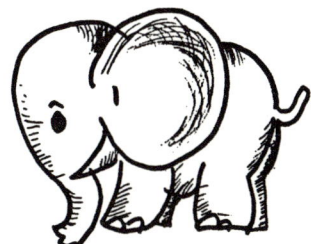

Procedure

Put the cornstarch and the baking soda in a saucepan and stir well. Mix in the water. Heat, stirring constantly, until the mixture reaches a slightly moist mashed-potato consistency.

Turn it out onto the plate and cover it with a damp cloth. When it is cool enough to handle, knead it like dough. Shape it as desired, or store it, tightly covered, for later use.

To shape Creative Clay, form it with the hands or roll it out to ¼" thickness and cut it with a knife or cookie cutter. If desired, it can be decorated with bits of clay, moistened and pressed in place. Pierce a hole near the edge for stringing pendants or ornaments.

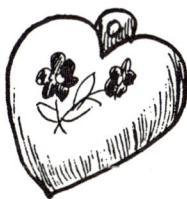 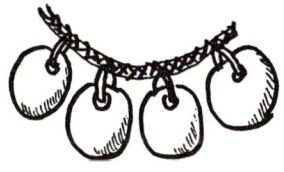 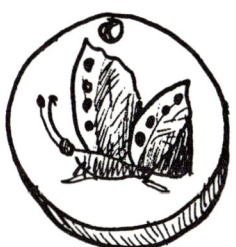

Let the items dry on a protected surface, or heat the oven to 350° F, turn it off, and leave the beads or other articles on a wire rack in the unlit oven for half an hour.

Creative Clay can be painted when dry with acrylics, water colors, poster paints, or felt-tip pens.

Brush with clear nail polish, varnish, or shellac for a protective coating.

Adaptations

People who need practice in measuring and food preparation can benefit from the experience of mixing this recipe. The pan holder referred to in Appendix C can be a help for some participants.

Those who need bilateral activities with light resistance will benefit from the kneading process.

A visually limited person can learn to measure by using specially marked cups available from the American Foundation for the Blind (see Appendix E) or can learn to measure with a set of graded standard measuring cups.

FLOWERS

Therapeutic Implications

The following projects involve primarily wrist and finger motion. The participant must be able to use scissors, twist wire, wrap tape, and (for the burlap flowers) draw threads. All three of these crafts require prehension and moderate strength in grasp and release. Wrist or elbow rotary action is required for the wrapping. These activities are good exercises where there is potential for increased hand strength or increased joint motion. They can be done best by someone who has a fair degree of dexterity in at least one hand. Precise cutting is needed for the fabric and cornhusk flowers. The assembly can be done with one hand, but is difficult at best. More resistance is encountered in making the fabric flowers, and greater strength is needed because the wire must be cut and twisted.

Although the selection and grouping of the fabric flowers is somewhat creative, the crafts are generally structured, routine, and repetitive. The steps are fairly simple and can be broken down into discrete units. Since the projects can be completed in a short time (one or two sessions, depending on the number made), they are good for participants whose attention span is short, or for those who need more immediate satisfaction.

People with limited visual acuity can probably do well with construction of the fabric flowers, where the wire provides good tactile feedback and a guide for completion.

Burlap Flowers

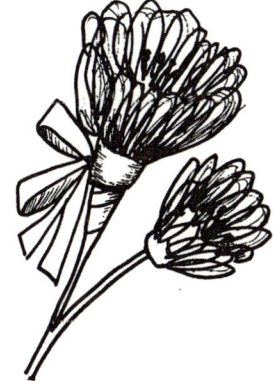

Materials

1. burlap in a variety of colors
2. pipe cleaners or flexible florist's wire (gauge 18-24)
3. green florist's tape
4. scissors
5. wire cutters
6. masking tape
7. white glue
8. ruler

Procedure

Cut the burlap to the desired flower size. For the initial instruction, 6″ × 4″ is recommended.

Leave a top and bottom margin of ½″ intact. Pull out all of the weft (6″ threads) between the top and bottom margins. Set these aside for use as stamens (centers) and as another variety of burlap flower. (See Figure 13-77.)

Spread a thin line of glue along the bottom margin of the burlap and let it get tacky. Press the top edge onto the glued surface, folding the original rectangle in half. (See Figures 13-78 and 13-79.)

Figure 13-77 Pulling Threads

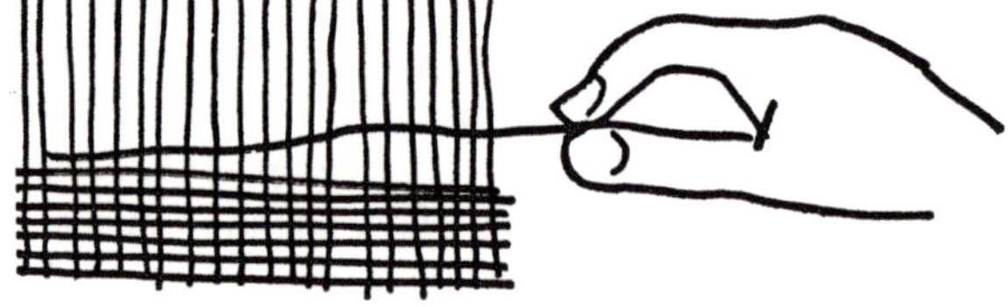

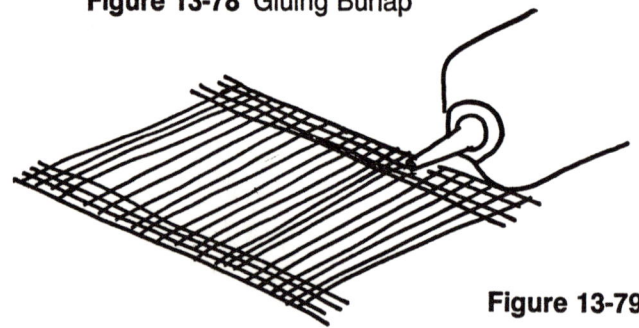

Figure 13-78 Gluing Burlap

Figure 13-79 Folded Burlap

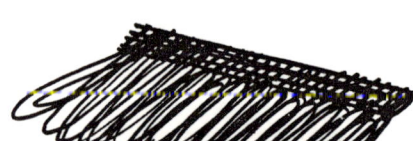

Figure 13-80 Rolling Flowers

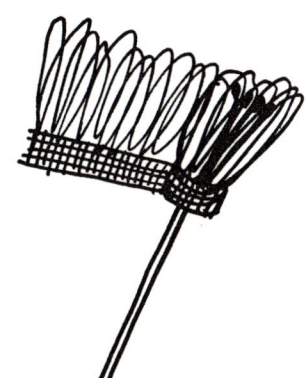

For the stamens, use about ten strands of ravelled threads of a contrasting color. Bend 1" of the wire stem over the center of the ten strands and twist it once or twice to secure the strands. Trim the strands to a uniform length of about 1."

For the flowers, place the stamens on the right edge of the glued rectangle, with their tops even with the top of the burlap. Roll tightly from right to left, keeping the top and bottom edges even. (See Figure 13-80.)

To complete the flower, start at the thick base just below the ravelled burlap and wrap the florist's tape tightly around the base and down the wire. This gives the stem a finished appearance.

Variations

These flowers can be made in any size, from miniatures (3" × 4") to larger than the 6" × 4" model. Extra threads saved from the raveling can be wired through the center to form another type of flower: hold the threads together, fold them in the center, and fasten them by bending one end of wire stem over them and twisting once or twice to secure them. Use florist's tape at the point above the secured threads and wrap it down the stem to finish. The center of this flower can be a glued on pom-pom, a button, or a spiral of pipe cleaner.

Burlap flowers can be made into corsages with ribbon and corsage pins, or arranged as bouquets with baby's breath or dried goldenrod, sprayed white, as a filler.

Bouquets can be designed for specific occasions (red, white, and blue for patriotic themes, green for St. Patrick's Day, yellow, orange, and brown for an autumn theme, etc.).

Adaptations

The burlap rectangle can be taped to the table with masking tape along the top and bottom edges. This will hold the fabric in place while the threads are pulled, and the width of the tape makes a perfect margin for the solid borders. Remove the tape before gluing the rectangle together.

Cornhusk Flowers

Materials

1. cornhusks
2. corn silk (optional)
3. wire, 18 gauge
4. strong thread
5. florist's tape
6. white glue
7. ruler
8. pencil
9. scissors
10. poppy pattern
11. leaf pattern
12. tracing paper
13. tray or shallow dish for soaking cornhusks

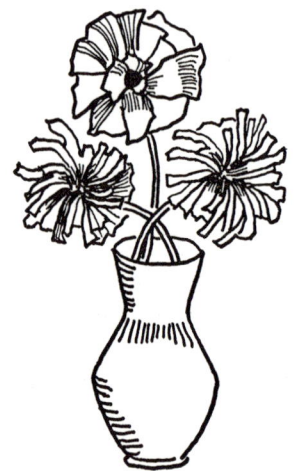

Procedure

Soak the husks in hot water to make them pliable. Work with the grain of the husks running vertically from top to bottom of the petal or leaf.

Shasta Daisy. Cut a wire 14" long for the stem and bend the top over to form a hook. Cover the bent end with a small piece of husk to conceal the end of the wire and to keep the finished flower from sliding off the stem.

From pieces of cornhusk 3" or 4" wide, shred or cut narrow strips to get enough for a full flower. Secure these strips in bunches around the prepared wire with strong thread. Work with wet cornhusks, so they will curl as they dry.

Wrap the stem with floral tape, adding leaves as you go.

Poppy. Enlarge and cut the patterns for the poppy petal and leaf. (See Figure 13-81 and Figures 13-46 to 13-49.) Cut six to ten poppy petals and three to four leaves for each flower, depending on the fullness desired. Bend and cover a 14" wire stem, as described for the daisy. Cut a piece of husk 2" wide. Gather the husk

Figure 13-81 Poppy Pattern

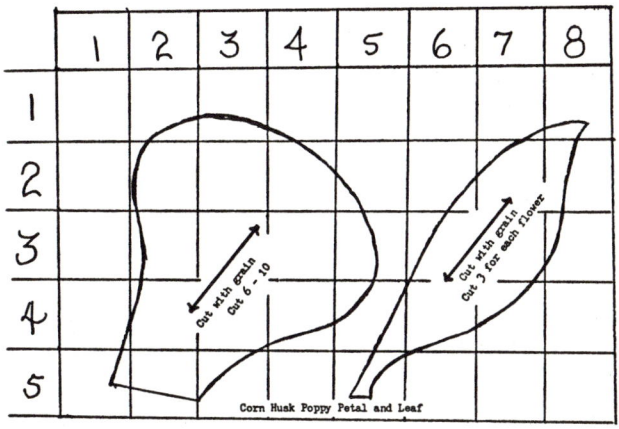

Corn Husk Poppy Petal and Leaf

around the hook end of the stem and secure it with strong thread to make the center for the poppy. Arrange the poppy petals around the covered hook, overlapping each petal, and secure them in place with wire or strong thread.

Cover the stem with florist's tape, adding poppy leaves along the stem.

To add depth to the finished flowers, glue a little corn silk to the centers.

Adaptations

The daisy construction can be simplified: Draw a 1" border at the bottom of the pieces (across the grain) of cornhusk, anchor the husk to the working surface with tape, and cut narrow strips up to the 1" line. This takes the place of the shredding process for those unable to cut completely through the husk. The special scissors listed in Appendix B can make the cutting easier for a one-handed person.

Tracing paper can be taped over the patterns to stabilize the work for a one-handed person.

Two one-handed persons can work on this project, or it can be a group effort with the members sharing parts of the project within their capabilities. The steps required are:

1. soaking and keeping the husks pliable
2. pattern tracing (after the pattern has been enlarged)
3. pattern cutting
4. cutting or shredding the husks for the daisy or cutting from patterns for the poppy and leaf
5. bending and covering the wire ends
6. adding the flowers (shreds or poppy petals)
7. wrapping the stems and adding the leaves

Fabric Flowers

Materials

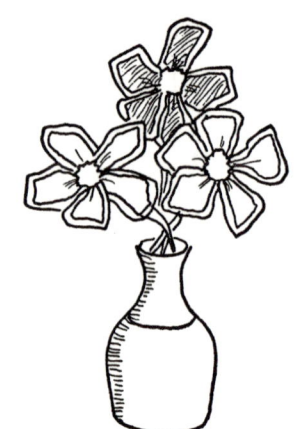

1. five 10" pipe cleaners for each flower
2. cotton fabric
3. white glue
4. floral stem wire, 10"
5. fine wire on a spool
6. florist's tape
7. small pom-poms for flower centers
8. scissors
9. wire cutter or old pair of scissors

Procedure

Cut the pipe cleaners into 10" lengths if the long ones are being used. To shape the petal, hold the pipe cleaner at a point 3" from one end. Curve the rest of the pipe cleaner to this point and twist the end to hold it securely in place.

Bend the 3" stem down at a right angle to form a loop. Apply glue to the top of the loop.

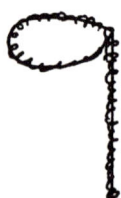

Invert the petal shape and place it on the right side of the fabric, pressing gently to make it adhere. Leave the 3" stem upright.

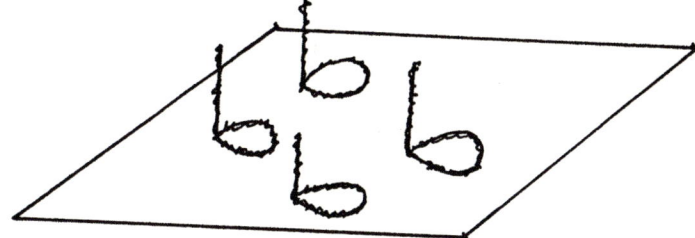

Let the parts dry thoroughly before continuing.

Cut away the fabric from around the outside edge of each loop to form the petals. Straighten out each pipe cleaner so the petal is in line with (rather than at a right angle to) the stem.

Bend a hook shape at one end of the 10'' floral stem wire (to keep the petals from slipping) and arrange the five petals around it. Hold them together with fine wire from the spool. Wrap the stem with florist's tape.

Glue a pom-pom, button, or cotton ball in the center of the flower.

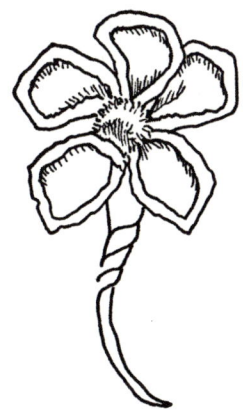

Variations

Pinking shears can be used to cut away the fabric from the petal rim.

Leaf shapes can be made by covering the petal shape with green fabric and leaving the pipe cleaner on the underside.

The pipe cleaner shape can be placed on the wrong side of the material to make a solid, untrimmed petal. A matching section of pipe cleaner can be coiled around a pencil, pulled into a loose coil, and used in the center of the flower.

Adaptations

A nail board can be clamped to the table to help form the pipe cleaner into the petal shape. (It is advisable to use pipe cleaners slightly longer than 10″ for this.)

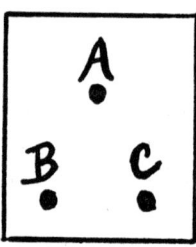

Bend the pipe cleaner in the middle and anchor it on nail A. Hold the two ends, wrap them around B and C, and twist the ends together and up. This provides the upright handle for gluing.

The petal shapes can be dipped in glue (which can be put on waxed paper or in a shallow dish for easier handling) and then placed on the fabric.

The excess fabric can be cut away with the special scissors listed in Appendix B.

Some assistance may be needed for assembling the petals and center stem. After the petals have been wired together, clamping the stem in a table vise will make it possible for the participant to wrap it with florist's tape.

NATURE MATERIALS

Therapeutic Implications

The crafts discussed in this chapter have in common the advantage of requiring little expense in materials and equipment. They work well for a group, and can also be done effectively by individuals. They are all relatively short term projects.

The primary physical tasks required are prehension and grasp-release use of the hand. They all necessitate some spatial planning, either visually or by touch. Those limited by fatigue should not be excluded from doing these light resistive projects.

Specific qualities of the individual projects are included here for instructor guidance in selection and phasing of the tasks.

Dried Arrangements

This is a light prehensile activity that can be done by those who have good hand dexterity but lack shoulder and elbow strength. It requires good vision or a good tactile sense for arrangement of materials.

Nature Craft Note Paper

Arranging dried leaves and flowers requires fine, light prehension. Tearing or cutting the paper has a resistive component, and is difficult with one hand. The final process of pressing requires grasp strength for handling the iron, exercises both elbow and shoulder muscles for lifting and sliding the iron. The fusion process should be limited to participants with good judgment and adequate sensation.

Nature Plaques

As plaques are best cut with an electric jigsaw, a staff member should prepare these. Sanding and finishing the base require little joint action but light grasp and minimal elbow or shoulder range. Fine dexterity and light prehension are necessary for placement of materials. Spatial planning is necessary for good results.

Pine Cone Angel

Handling the materials for this project requires light prehension and a fair degree of dexterity. Fine dexterity is needed to paint the facial features.

Pine Cone Wreath

This is an excellent project for those with light grasp ability. For the visually impaired, sorting of the various sized cones and other materials can be good training for tactile discrimination. The visually limited can be guided to feel spaces where they cannot see them.

Pomander Ball

The pressure required to place the cloves necessitates good prehensile strength. Covering all the space on the orange requires fine dexterity. It is repetitive and easily learned, but those with sensory deficits in the hand would find this a difficult craft.

Sand Terrarium

This project lends itself to more creativity. The concept of layering and sculpturing the sand requires abstract reasoning, making it difficult for those who have limited mental abilities. It is a light grasp activity, requiring some elbow-shoulder motion. Good vision is essential, since the results cannot be felt.

Stone Painting

Creativity can also be stimulated through this project, although stencils or transfer patterns could be used. Dexterity and light prehension are essential for this precision painting task.

Dried Arrangements

Materials

1. white glue
2. clear spray
3. Styrofoam in small pieces
4. waxed paper for working surface
5. paper towels for clean-up
6. scissors
7. assorted dried weeds, cones, seed pods, and grasses
8. pieces of bark or driftwood
9. soft covering materials, such as moss, to camouflage the Styrofoam

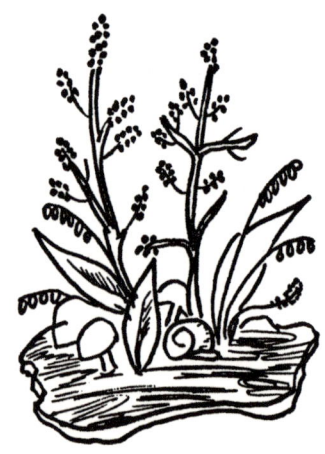

Procedure

Glue small pieces of Styrofoam to the bark or driftwood to form the base for the arrangement. Allow it to dry for several hours.

Arrange the dried grasses, pods, and other materials, inserting the stems into the styrofoam, just as fresh flowers would be arranged. Dip the stems into the glue before inserting them to make them more secure. Camouflage the Styrofoam with moss or other soft materials and finish by applying clear acrylic spray.

Ikebana is an appealing technique for dried arrangements. This is a Japanese design in which the placement of the various materials has significance. The three main elements are heaven, man, and earth. Heaven is the tallest element, standing in the center. For man, use the same material but place it a little lower than heaven and to the left. For earth, use the same material as for heaven and man, and place it a little lower than man and to the right. These elements form a triangle. Other materials are added along the above basic lines: mountains, a little lower than heaven; woman, a little lower than man; water, lower than earth.

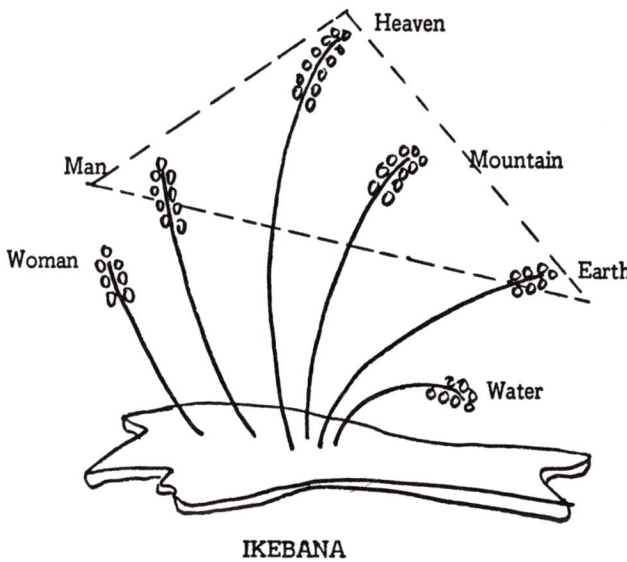

IKEBANA

Adaptations

An anchoring medium, such as florist's clay, may be needed. Some assistance may be necessary for cutting or pulling apart the dried materials.

Nature Craft Note Paper

Materials

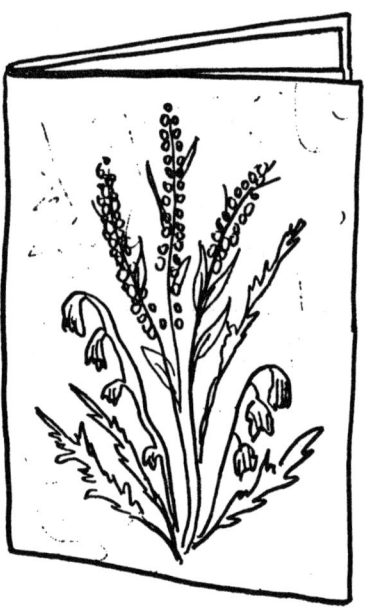

1. scissors
2. white glue diluted half water, half glue
3. brush for glue
4. electric iron
5. masking tape
6. cleansing tissues, pastel shades
7. waxed paper
8. brown paper bags or newspapers
9. blotters, toweling, or any absorbent material
10. dried pressed flowers, weeds, or leaves
11. 20 lb. weight typing paper, or cover stock, 8½" × 11"

Procedure

Cut the paper in half to measure 5½" × 8½." Fold it in half to get a note card size of 4¼" × 5½." (This is the standard size for note paper, and can be matched with envelopes from stationery stores.)

Open the folded note paper so that it lies flat, right side up. Place a sheet of waxed paper over it, allowing generous margins. (The note paper, at this point in the procedure, is just a guide so that the dried arrangement can be placed suitably. It is not to be glued.) Using the right half of the note paper as a guide, arrange the dried material. (See Figure 13-82.)

Place a single sheet of tissue over the arrangement, and brush the entire area of the tissue with diluted white glue. Figure 13-83 shows the layering of the materials in preparation for the glue application.

The note paper can be removed and used again as a guide for the next arrangement.

Set the project aside to dry, or dry in a slow oven (225° F) for approximately twenty minutes. When dry, place the waxed paper arrangement inside a brown paper bag or between sheets of newspaper, waxed side up, and press with a warm iron (set for "synthetics") to melt the wax.

Figure 13-82 First Step

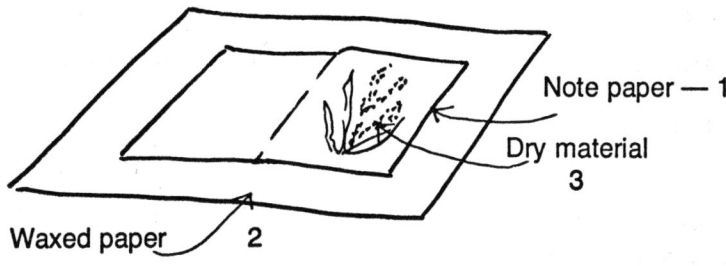

Figure 13-83 Second Step

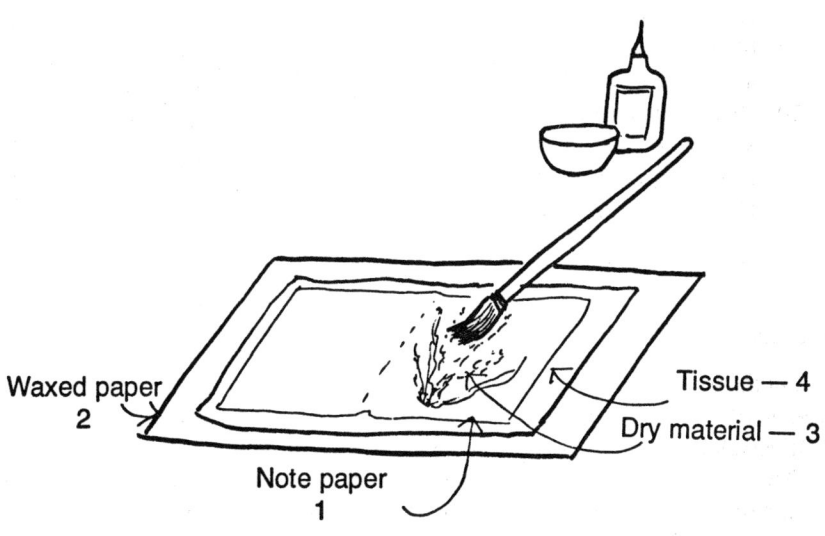

Align the arrangement on the stationery and carefully tear or cut the edges, using a ruler for tearing to give a deckle-edge effect. Fold the waxed arrangement in half, apply glue on the folded crease of note paper, and insert it into the crease of the waxed arrangement sheet. Note: Some brands of tissue come in four pastel shades per box, and give a choice of colors.

Variations

Purchased blank note paper, in colors with matching envelopes, can be used.
Book marks, gift tags, and bridge tallies are other items that can be made using this process.

Adaptations

For those with mild coordination problems, or the use of only one hand, the waxed paper and the tissue can be anchored to the table with masking tape. Assistance may be needed with cutting or tearing in the final stage. A paper cutter, if available, will allow some people to work independently if they weight the paper down while cutting. A T-square or board with corner guard may be helpful in assisting with the folding.

Nature Plaques

Materials

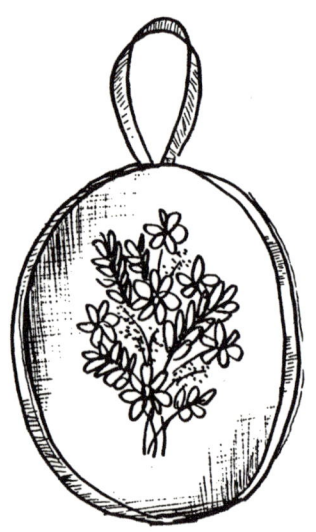

1. jigsaw
2. sandpaper, fine grade
3. clear varnish spray, non-toxic
4. waxed paper
5. white glue
6. scissors
7. lightweight pine, thin plywood, or other easily cut wood, 5" × 7"
8. dried flowers, weeds, and seedpods
9. spray enamel, in various colors
10. small strawflowers from florist
11. cording or ribbon for edging and hanger

Procedure

Gather and spray with enamel a variety of weeds and seedpods that have dried thoroughly. When picking natural material for this purpose, include some long weeds or flowers, because they can be used for large plaques or cut into shorter pieces.

Trace an oval or round shape on the wood and cut it out with a jigsaw. Sand the surface and edges of the wood.

Working on a waxed paper covered surface, place the dried materials in one corner and pour a small amount of glue in the other corner. If the plaque is placed in the center of the work space, the necessary materials will then be handy. Dip each piece of dried material into the glue and arrange it on the plaque. Allow the glue to dry thoroughly, then spray the entire plaque with clear varnish. This will set the dried arrangement firmly in place and give a solid finish to the plaque.

When the varnish is dry, use cording or ribbon around the edges, as shown in Figure 13-84. Apply glue all around the edge of the plaque. When it becomes tacky, start at the bottom and wrap the ribbon or cording around the edge, pressing it firmly into the glued surface. At the bottom, cut the ribbon carefully so that the joining is inconspicuous. The ribbon or cording should not be wider than the thickness of the plaque.

Cut a 3'' piece of ribbon and apply a spot of glue to one end. Press the other end on top of the glue, giving it one twist before gluing, so that the ribbon makes an open loop that will hang easily over a nail. (See Figure 13-85.)

Put a spot of glue on the top of the joined loop, and lay the plaque on it at the best point of attachment.

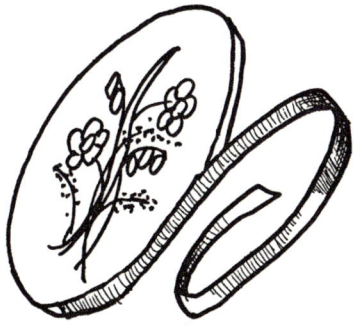

Figure 13-84 Edging

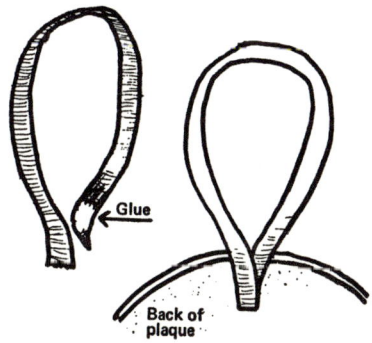

Figure 13-85 Fastening the Hanger

Variations

Sizes can vary from miniature to large, depending on materials available and intended uses. Assorted sizes and shapes of precut wood bases are available at most hobby or craft stores.

Adaptations

For the person with the use of only one hand, anchor the waxed paper to the working surface with masking tape, use a C-clamp to hold either a sanding block or the plaque in place for sanding, and assist with cutting the dried materials if necessary. (However, most dried materials can be snapped apart easily with the fingers of one hand.)

Pine Cone Angels

Materials

1. scissors
2. white glue
3. brushes for glue
4. sharp knife
5. medium size pine cones
6. acorns with caps
7. milkweed pods

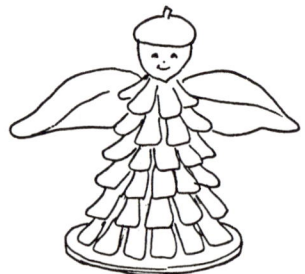

Procedure

Stand the pine cone stem-side up. (Some trimming may be necessary to make it flat on the bottom.) Glue the acorn to the top of the cone for a head. The cap will make a little hat.

Split the pod and remove the silk. Each side of the pod will make a wing. Glue on the two wings, and allow ample time for drying.

Paint on features and add anything that might come to mind. Try adding a halo, some glitter, and touches of color. Then put the angel on a base, add a loop for hanging, or perhaps add the figure to a grouping in a shadow box.

Adaptations

Allow the glue to get tacky so that a minimal amount of pressure is needed to hold the added pieces in place.

Use florist's clay to anchor the pine cone to a base while working on it.

Pine Cone Wreath

Materials

1. heavy cardboard or lightweight plywood
2. scissors
3. masking tape or wood-tone contact paper
4. white glue
5. assorted pine cones and fir, pine, and spruce branches
6. small piece of wire (about 5") for hanging loop

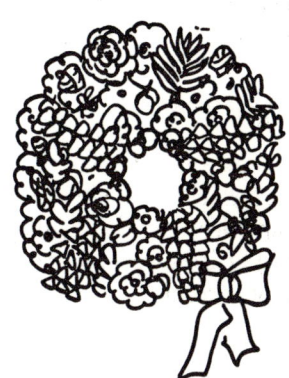

Procedure

Cut a 10" circle from heavy cardboard or lightweight plywood. Cut out a 3" or 4" diameter hole within this circle.

Wrap the edges of the cardboard with masking tape or cover the surface with contact paper. Attach a small wire loop to the back by pushing the wire from front to back in two places and twisting the wire ends together in back.

Pull several pine cones apart to provide a supply of bracts. Glue the bracts close together around the outer and inner circles and then fill in the remaining area with the other materials.

Dip the pine cones in glue, or spot-glue the base with a brush, and apply the cones and other materials. Place the large pine cones (red or white pine) in position first, as a base and to establish a design. Then add the medium sized cones (Douglas fir, Eastern spruce). Use pine cone bracts as edging. Use all types of cones, and pine cones cut in half through the middle, to build up and fill in. The first large cones can be wired on for better anchoring, but gluing can be done throughout. (Be sure the base cones are well secured before adding layers.)

For finishing, the smaller materials can consist of tiny cones, any dried weed or flower, acorns, and nuts. White pine cones can be cut into sections to form rosettes for finishing or to fill in spots.

After the glue is thoroughly dry, spray the wreath with several coats of acrylic spray (crystal). A light spraying of gold with some glitter added can also be used. Dry thoroughly between each coat. (It may be advisable to have the staff do this.)

Add a colored bow at the top.

Variations

- Miniature wreaths with the smaller materials are attractive.
- A small Christmas tree shape cut from cardboard and covered with smaller pieces of material and pine cones can be hung or made free-standing.
- Small sprays of branches can be tied together with wire and cones and finished off with a red or green ribbon bow.
- The branches can be sprayed, or left green, and the pine cones can be sprayed with gold or silver paint.
- Small arrangements can be glued to a wooden base, then sprayed with acrylic. (Add a hook at the back for hanging.)

Adaptations

The pine cones can be clamped in a woodworking vise so the participant can cut or tear off the bracts.

Small pine cones can be substituted for the bracts to cover the edges of the cardboard.

It helps to have a quantity of precut materials handy so only the dipping and arranging will need to be done and the participants can work independently.

Pomander Balls

Materials

1. 1 thick-skinned orange
2. 3 oz. whole cloves
3. 1 tbs. ground cinnamon
4. 1 tsp. orrisroot (from supermarket or pharmacy)
5. ribbon

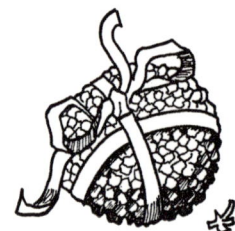

Procedure

Wash the orange and wipe dry. Using a skewer or nail to start the holes, insert whole cloves in the skin, covering the entire surface.

Mix cinnamon and orrisroot and put a heaping teaspoon in a small bag with the orange. Shake the bag to coat the orange well. Wrap the orange loosely or place it in a foil-covered tray or basket.

Store in a dry place until the orange shrinks and hardens (in three to four weeks), turning it every few days.

Tie the pomander ball with colored ribbon and hang it in a closet or storage bag.

Adaptations

Place the orange on a stabilized nail (see *Adaptations* under **Mexican Jewelry and Dolls**) to secure it when working. It can be turned around on the wooden base as the surface is covered.

People with visual handicaps may have trouble getting the cloves close enough together; if so, the project can be done as a group effort, with a sighted person doing the final filling in.

To get the cloves into the holes, a visually limited person should hold the nail in the proper spot with one hand while placing a clove in the hole with the other. (This is of course impossible for someone who has the use of only one hand.) However, some persons can compensate if they have a good sense of discrimination. Putting the cloves on a white or light-colored background or dish will help.

Sand Terrarium

Figure 13-86 Water Mountain Scene

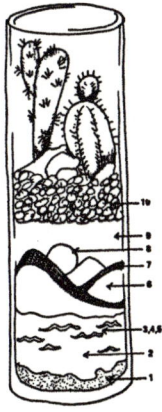

Materials

1. planter, glass jar, or other clear glass or plastic container
2. spoon
3. sand-setting tool (knitting needle, skewer, or toothpick)
4. funnel
5. terrarium sand in a variety of colors
6. beach sand or potting soil

Procedure

To practice: Pour a packet of sand in a glass. Poke the point of the tool into the sand, pressing firmly against the glass. (See A and B.) Turn the tool around and do the same thing with the flat or round end. (See C.)

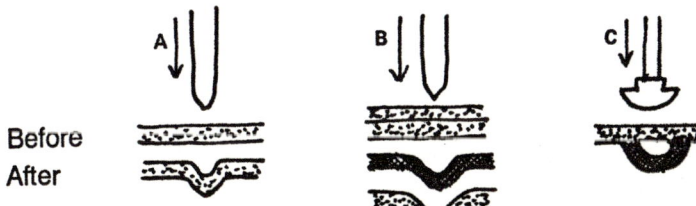

Making a Water Mountain Scene

(Steps are numbered as in Figure 13-86.)

1. Pour in a layer of natural brown sand, making uneven mounds. This is the beach foreground. Shape it with the flat end of the tool.
2. Pour about ½" of blue sand on top of the natural sand to represent water.
3. With a spoon, carefully pour ⅛" of white sand on the blue. Drop sand against the glass at several spots.
4. Using the pointed end of the tool, poke the white sand gently to form whitecaps on the blue water. Work slowly. (Fine-grain sand stays in place well.)
5. Add ¼" of blue sand. Repeat step No. 4 for more whitecaps.
6. Pour uneven mounds of red or brown sand to form mountains. Use the flat end of the tool to shape the sides and peaks.
7. To make separating lines, use natural brown sand.
8. Pour yellow or orange sand between the mountain peaks against the glass. Form the sun with the tool point.
9. Using a spoon, add a level layer of light blue to form the sky.
10. For plants, use house plant soil mixed with 1/3 sand. Decorate the top with rocks and gravel or with colored sand.

Making an Indian Sand Painting

(Steps are numbered as in Figure 13-87.)

1. Pour a layer of any colored sand into the container.
2. Shape the sand with the flat end of the tool. Add some contrasting colored sand.
3. Repeat with different sands to create the design.
4. To make layer penetrations as in No. 3 and No. 4, use the pointed end of the tool. Quickly jab it down and up in a jerking motion through as many layers as desired, holding the tool firmly against the glass.
5. Plant the plants as in step No. 10 for the water mountain scene. To make colored sand, use fine grade masonry sand from a lumber yard, and mix it with wet tempera (only the tempera should be wet). Allow it to dry thoroughly before using it for sand painting.

Variations

Use a small plastic drinking glass with a minimum of three or four colors of sand as a beginning project. A single miniature plant can be imbedded in a layer of soil covered with pebbles or small stones. This is a good short-term project.

The sharing of sand and tools can make this a good group project for socializing.

Figure 13-87 Indian Sand Painting

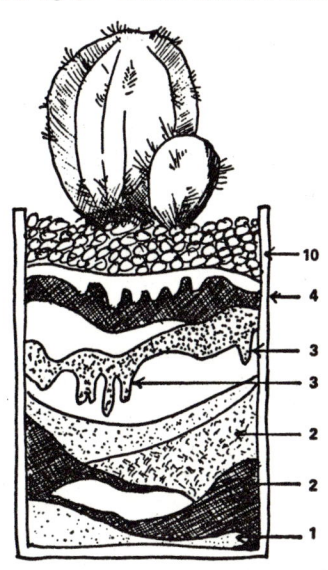

Adaptations

Pouring sand from an envelope might be difficult with one hand. If so, transfer the sand to a dish from which it can be scooped with a spoon, or put the sand in a pill bottle for pouring.

Colored sand is not necessary for the center of the container; ordinary soil and plain sand can be built up in the center as the design progresses up the sides of the container.

Stone Painting

Materials

1. white glue or epoxy cement
2. paints: acrylic, enamel, or latex
3. brushes
4. felt-tip markers, indelible
5. waxed paper and paper towels
6. clear spray enamel or polyurethane varnish
7. assorted stones, especially smooth beach stones
8. interesting bark or driftwood

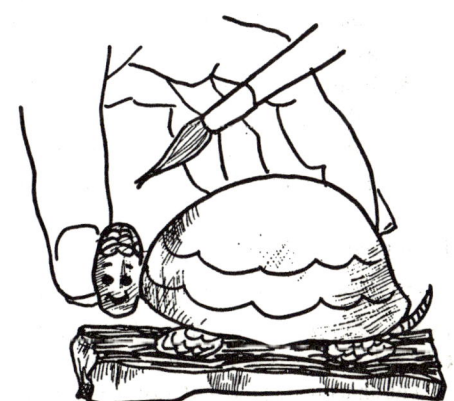

Procedure

Wash and dry the stones, shells, and driftwood. Work on a waxed paper surface.

Frequently the shape of the stone will suggest an animal, figure, or free-form design. With a felt-tip marker or paint, draw features or designs on the stones and fill in with chosen colors. Owls, ladybugs, ducks, and turtles come most easily to mind as the stones are sorted. After the figure or other object has been painted and varnished, it can be placed on a piece of driftwood or other base.

Variations

Pin or earring backings can be glued to ladybugs and other small painted stones to make ornamental pins, earrings, or other stone jewelry.

Adaptations

For the person with the use of only one hand, anchor the stones and driftwood to the working surface with florist's clay or masking tape.

HORTICULTURE

Therapeutic Implications

This medium can be used by all ages. It is enjoyable to watch a grapefruit seed sprout and grow into a beautiful plant. Pineapple tops root easily, as do avocado pits, sweet potato eyes, peas, and beans. (See *Plants from the Kitchen*.) Elaborate equipment is not necessary, and jars, old cups, and bowls discarded from the kitchen make interesting containers.

It is creative; a real garden outside, or a windowsill garden inside, gives a person an opportunity to produce something of beauty and a source of food. Starting plants from seeds (see *Egg Carton Garden*) or from cuttings gives hours of pleasure and satisfaction. It provides an opportunity to share an interest, and builds self-esteem. Caring for a collection of house plants can become an engrossing hobby.

Gro-lights and thermostatically controlled soil bed units offer a sophisticated means of growing and propagating plants. A small greenhouse with wheelchair-height trays allows chair-bound people to participate. Opportunities are endless, depending on space, money, and the participants' abilities.

Visually limited persons can work easily with sturdy plants. A fragrance garden or a windowsill garden with aromatic herbs can stimulate their interest.

Those who are limited in hearing or speech have a means of creative communication.

Windowsill gardening or table-level plantings provide useful outlets for those who have limited endurance because of cardiac problems; they can participate at their own speed, resting between each activity. Potting can be done even by those who cannot sit, because it can be accomplished from a prone position if the participant has adequate hand use.

Participants with joint disease will find that table-level pottings produce little stress; however, working in damp soil can cause additional stiffness in some people. Garden gloves may be enough to prevent this, but they tend to limit joint action.

Since planting requires specific steps, it is useful for improving concentration and planning abilities.

Some people with respiratory problems may not be able to participate fully in a horticulture program, depending upon the plants involved. For example, asthmatics and those with allergies may react adversely if exposed to certain odors in planting. This is particularly true in projects involving dried flowers and weeds.

Egg Carton Gardens

Materials

1. popsicle sticks or craft sticks
2. paper cups
3. large spoon
4. aluminum foil
5. packages of seeds (herbs for indoors; vegetables for transplanting)
6. soil
7. egg cartons (paper pulp; no plastic)

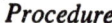

Procedure

Spoon soil into the egg spaces, then follow the directions on the seed packages for the proper depth to plant the seeds. Cover the seeds lightly with soil, and carefully water them by sprinkling with a spoon or using a plant sprayer or mister.

Cover the discarded egg carton top with aluminum foil and use it as a tray. This will catch the leakage when watering, and make a good base for the garden.

If this is a group activity, print participants' names on the popsicle or craft sticks, with the kind of seed and date of planting.

Variations

Small butter tubs or other shallow containers can be used in the same way.

Adaptations

It may be necessary to line the tray for one-handed participant.

Plants from the Kitchen

Materials

1. flower pots or containers
2. soil (different kinds for different plants)
3. spray bottle or mister
4. cord
5. knife
6. pits of citrus fruits or avocados, pineapple top, or potato or carrot cuttings

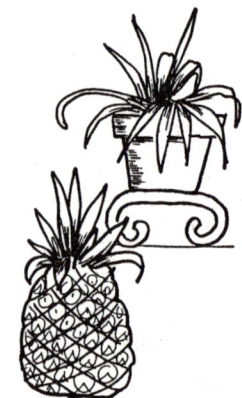

Procedure

"Fun gardens" can be created from the seeds of citrus fruits and cuttings from some common vegetables.

Citrus Fruits. The secret is to plant the seeds immediately after cutting open the fruit. They should be sown just deep enough to be completely covered by soil. The soil must be kept moist, and plants need frequent misting or spraying and good sun. Although citrus plants raised this way frequently have blossoms, they are not likely to produce fruit if kept inside.

Avocado Trees. To get an avocado pit started, soak it in water for a day or two to soften the outer casing. Peel off any remaining skin and plant the pit, with its pointed end up, in humus-enriched potting soil, leaving half the pit above soil level. With a large pot (7'' or 8'' across), frequent watering, feeding, and some sun, an avocado tree can attain ceiling height in a fairly short time.

Pineapple Plants. Cut off the top of a fully ripe pineapple an inch or two below the leaves. Trim away the soft fruit in the top but not the hard inner core. Pluck out the small outer leaves to expose the white and bright-green inner leaves. Then prepare a potting mixture of peat moss mixed with fine gravel and sand, and place the pineapple top on the dampened mixture. Secure it there with cord or masking tape. Next mist the pineapple top with warm water and place it in a good light until it roots, after which the plant will require only a few hours of sun a day. Water only the center cup of the plant, and keep the potting mixture moist.

Potato Plant. Cut off a section of the potato, say a quarter of it, making sure it contains at least one eye. Plant it deep enough so that all of the potato except the eye is completely covered.

Carrot Plant. Carrot tops can be planted like potatoes, and will grow lacy, fern-like foilage. Leave some of the carrot attached when planting.

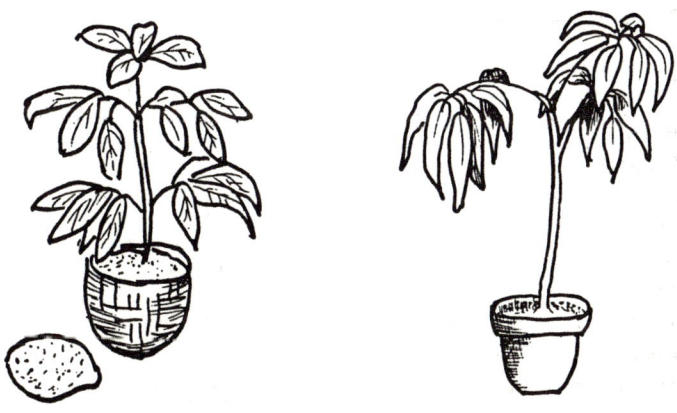

Drying Grasses, Flowers, Cones, and Seedpods

Flowers, Leaves, and Grasses

Collect the plants in midday when they contain the least amount of moisture. Press them between pages of heavy telephone books or other large books, or any absorbent paper, and put weights on top.

Allow enough time (approximately one week) so that all the moisture is gone and the flowers and grasses are easily freed from the pages. They will be fragile, and any not to be used within a few days should be replaced (for storage) in the books.

Some plants that can be hung upside down until dry include:

- everlasting flowers (straw flowers)
- poor man's money
- chives
- cockscomb
- yarrow
- goldenrod

Pods and Cones

Bake cones, acorns, nuts, and seedpods in a 200° F oven for approximately 30 minutes before using or storing them. This dries them and prevents mildew or fungal growth, and kills any bugs that may be hidden in them. Store them in a dry place.

Shells, Stones, and Driftwood

These are great additions to dried arrangements. They should be washed well before storing and use.

Refer to the *Crafts* section of the Bibliography for more information.

WOODWORKING

Therapeutic Implications

Woodworking is easily adapted for many individual needs. It can be expanded to meet the therapeutic goals of increasing function, or can be simplified to accommodate the limitations of severe handicaps.

Its value as a functional exercise is that it provides a means of increasing muscle strength, coordination, and range of motion. It is resistive by nature of its raw materials. Projects can easily be placed higher or farther away for sanding by the use of adjustable vises, slant boards, or adjustable tables. Weighted sanders make sanding more difficult and thus more resistive. Work can be positioned to one side to increase the range in shoulder-side reaching.

Coordination can be improved through assembly of pieces, gluing, and nailing, as well as by the use of tools. Smaller projects requiring finer work offer possibilities for improving dexterity; for example, putting together a model airplane or doll's house furniture requires more dexterity than assembling a child's bench.

This craft is a structured activity. Certain steps must be followed to complete the project successfully, and this encourages better organizing and sequencing. The projects can easily be broken down for those who are able to follow only one-level directions.

The projects require a broad range of physical and mental abilities. Those who are less limited may be able to make their own patterns and do their own sanding, sawing, assembling, and finishing. Those with more limited abilities can function best with precut projects. A severely impaired person can often do sanding and finishing, but may be unable to assemble components without a great deal of assistance. This illustrates the value of having available a variety of one-piece projects, such as chopping boards, decoupage bases, and hanging boards. It is best to have graph paper, measuring tools, and cardboards for patterns on hand to encourage people to make their own patterns. Graph paper is helpful for laying out pieces or for enlarging designs from printed patterns in books or magazines. (See *Enlarging or Reducing a Design*, under *Stitchery*.) Rulers and squares are necessary for making sure that the pattern is sized right. The graph pattern can be transferred to cardboard or to x-ray film if the project has potential for further use.

Since most of the projects are useful, they provide natural motivation for involvement. If participants cannot use the items produced, they may be motivated to make gifts for family or friends. Other projects, such as the checkerboard, can provide another incentive as something of worth to the activity center. If the products are salable, the producers may be motivated by being allowed to participate in deciding what will be purchased with the profits. Many people enjoy doing things for other community programs, such as making wooden toys for a nursery school.

The variety of finishing materials makes possible many variations. For example, a visually impaired person may have difficulty seeing whether a varnish finish has covered a piece adequately, but the use of bright paint will make it more visible. Rub-on wax may be the best finish in this instance, since the application of several coats will usually cover the piece.

For the person limited to the use of one hand, pieces can be stabilized by clamping. Often a dexterous person can learn to position C-clamps independently by putting the screw post on top of the piece, instead of underneath, and screwing the clamp to the approximate depth before tightening it on the work piece. C-clamps and vises can be padded with leather or moleskin to prevent pressure marks on wood.

Assembling pieces is more difficult. Pre-nailing is helpful for everyone. A nail can be started by making a hole with an awl to stabilize the nail while hammering it through one piece until it just penetrates the bottom surface. If each piece is then glued and allowed to dry, the final nailing can be done without clamping. Physical assistance will, of course, be required for some people. It is helpful to stabilize the nail with needle-nose pliers to prevent injury to the person assisting. This also keeps the nail straight.

The therapeutic objective for those whose limitations are complicated by a visual field impairment is to have them learn to compensate for the deficit by turning the head. Because some people lack the awareness to do this, one must position the project within the good visual field. This may mean positioning high or low, in addition to right or left, depending on the nature of the deficit. Although testing is useful in evaluating a person's deficit, the supervising staff member can usually determine the position of best visibility by observing the person in action (e.g., some people sand only one side of a board, being unaware of the other).

Perceptual and sensory deficits call for more structure. Assistance may be necessary in projects such as drawing lines where nails are to be placed or putting masking tape or tongue depressors along a predetermined nail line as a guide. People may become confused if too many tools or work pieces are put in front of them.

A person with good sensation but a visual impairment may have to be oriented, verbally and by touch, to the tool positions and work pieces. If the problem is poor sensation, visual cues will be needed.

Woodworking appeals to most men, and experience has shown that the camaraderie of an all-male group has its benefits. However, it is an activity that should not be limited by sex. Many women enjoy it because of the useful household items it can produce and because they are often manually dexterous.

Since this craft usually involves pounding, pushing, and exertion of gross muscle strength, it is a useful outlet for someone who harbors frustration and anger. Larger pieces are usually best for those who need a constructive outlet for their emotions. Fine work, such as doll's house furniture, might prove frustrating. Care should be taken with a person who exhibits depression, because sharp tools are always potentially dangerous.

For those who are physically and mentally capable of independence, it is important to allow for a greater range of projects. It is helpful to have on hand books and craft magazines that contain ideas for new projects. Describing a problem or a need in the facility may give a person the incentive to create a design (such as a magazine or book rack) to fill the need. If a participant wants to make something for the home that extends beyond the materials available, a family member may be willing to provide the materials or help defray the cost.

Precautions

- For those with sensory problems, it is important to be cautious with the use of sharp tools and cleaning materials. Oil-base paints and wood stains can burn people without their being aware of it.
- For those with respiratory problems, exposure to sawdust, paints, and stains may be inadvisable. Adequate ventilation is essential.
- The use of any tools should be supervised carefully, because tools can slip and become hazardous.
- Electrical tools should be used only by people, including staff members, who have been instructed in their safe handling. Proper wiring and insulation are essential. Safety goggles should always be worn, and the working space for tool users should be unobstructed. Official health and safety guidelines must be followed. If there are no qualified instructors in the program, woodwork instructors from other local craft programs or schools might be recruited to teach. Anyone prone to seizures should never be permitted to use electrical tools.

Setting up a Shop

Working with wood can be as simple or as complex as space, equipment, and participant abilities permit.

Kits that require only sanding or painting, gluing, and assembling can be worked into almost any program. However, the satisfaction and therapy derived from starting a project with the raw material and carrying it through to its final stage provide an incentive and source of satisfaction that are not always possible with kits.

The following list shows the equipment and materials needed for a basic workshop for making many attractive and useful projects.

Equipment
- handsaw or jigsaw
- C-clamps
- portable swivel vises
- hammers, lightweight
- brads, assorted sizes (¾''-1¼'')
- nails, assorted
- T-square
- carpenter's square
- ruler
- yardstick
- gimlet or awl
- needle-nose pliers

Materials
- softwood, such as white pine
- clear plywood
- Masonite
- masking tape
- clear varnish, non-toxic
- varnish stain
- wood scraps from lumber yard
- sandpaper, assorted grades (fine and medium for pre-cut projects)
- sanding blocks
- rags
- aprons

- pre-cut wood projects (see Appendix C)
- newspapers
- paints, assorted colors, latex*
- white glue, water soluble
- Sobo glue for outdoor projects
- brushes, assorted sizes
- turpentine
- throw-away plastic gloves (surgical gloves work nicely)
- metal container with lid for disposal of rags and paper used with oil-base stain and paint, marked according to safety codes

For a more versatile shop, some of the following equipment can be added:

- miter box and back saw
- electric drill and assorted bits, including countersink bit
- standard screwdriver (short handled is best)
- plane
- flathead screws (¾"-1½" long, No. 5-8)
- jigsaw, hand, electric
- jigsaw, table, electric
- rachet screwdriver
- surform planes, short and long
- workbenches (see *Woodworking Adaptations at the end of this section.*)
- plastic wood and thinner

A shop thus equipped can make useful equipment for its own use and for other departments.

---

*The first coat should be flat to seal the wood; the second coat should be semi-gloss (gloss is very shiny).

Pegboard, showing tool arrangement and numbering for color coding.

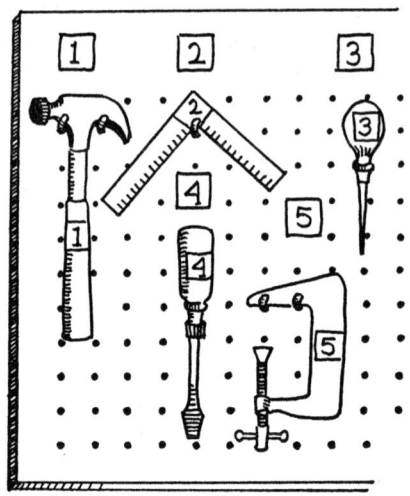

Hangboard

Materials

1. hammer
2. nail or gimlet to start cup hooks
3. brush for varnish
4. quick-dry varnish
5. white glue
6. glue brushes
7. sandpaper
8. piece of wood, approximately 5" × 10"
9. six cup hooks
10. pictures cut from greeting cards, calendars, etc. (on fairly heavy paper)
11. picture hooks
12. turpentine to clean brushes

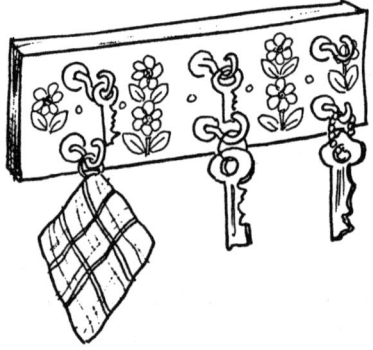

Procedure

Sand, then stain or paint, the wood. Put nail holes in the boards where the hooks are to be placed. Glue the pictures to the board, arranging them around the holes where the hooks will be. Use the glue sparingly and allow it to dry thoroughly.

Coat the top and sides with varnish, covering the pictures too.

Screw the cup hooks into the holes and attach picture hooks to the back of the board for hanging.

Hanging Herb Garden

Materials

1. saw
2. hammer
3. finishing nails, 1″
4. white glue
5. ten or twelve wood lath strips, 1½″ × 14″
6. two plywood half circles from a 7″ diameter circle
7. four screw eyes, ¼″
8. wood stain
9. four yards macramé cord
10. aluminum foil to line basket
11. sphagnum moss and potting soil
12. herb seeds (parsley, marjoram, oregano, etc.)

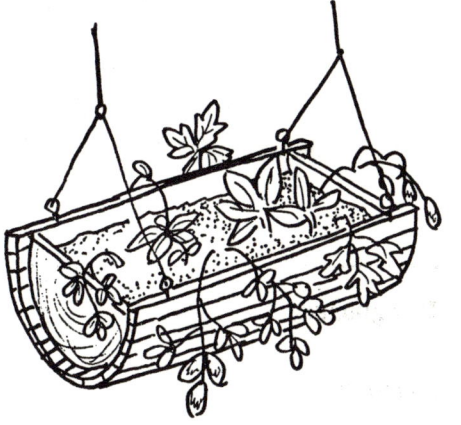

The liner for the basket is optional. Heavy-duty aluminum foil or lightweight aluminum can be used.

Procedure

Check to see that there are enough wood lath strips to go completely around the semicircular wood ends, close enough to touch each other. Glue and nail the strips to the ends, cradle fashion.

Attach screw eyes to the four ends of the planter, 1″ in from the corners. Run macramé cord underneath both ends of the planter and through the screw eyes. Tie square knots and a decorative pattern about 14″ above the planter.

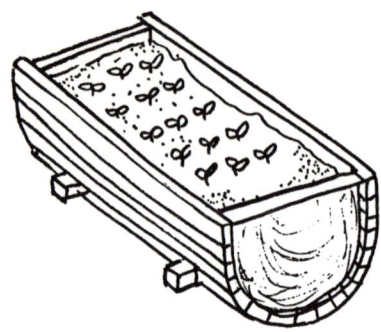

Line the planter with sphagnum moss and fill it to ¼'' from the top with potting soil. Plant herb seeds according to the package directions.

Hang in a window where there is strong light. (Direct sunlight is not necessary.)

Hanging Planter

Materials

1. vise
2. crosscut saw
3. sandpaper, medium and fine
4. sanding block
5. nails, 1'' common or finishing
6. hammer
7. white glue
8. plywood, ¼''
9. pine stripping, ¾'' × ¾''
10. wood stain
11. rags for wiping off stain
12. chain or heavy cord
13. four screw eyes

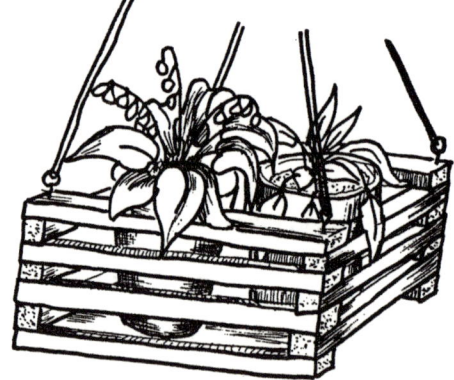

Procedure

Cut a 9'' square from the plywood. Cut fourteen 9'' lengths from the pine strips. Sand them well, stain, and let dry.

Glue and nail in place, on opposite sides of the 9'' plywood square, two pieces of stripping. This is the footing and base of the planter.

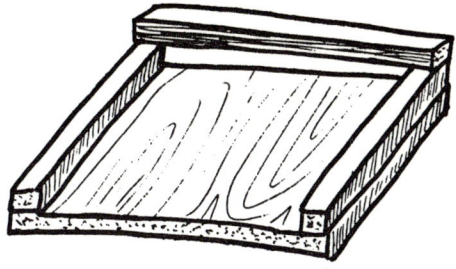

Glue and nail in place the next two strips on the opposite sides of the 9" square. The ends rest on the first pair of strips. Continue building up the sides with each pair resting on the strips below, in alternating layers.

Add the screw eyes to each of the four corners of the last pieces of stripping, and attach the chain or heavy cord for hanging.

Variations

Other kinds of wood can be used, and the size of the planter can vary. A miniature one to hold small flower pots would be attractive.

Paint can be used instead of varnish.

Playing Card Holder

Materials

1. jigsaw
2. plane
3. pine, ¾" or ½"
4. sandpaper
5. varnish or stain
6. cardboard
7. vise
8. glue

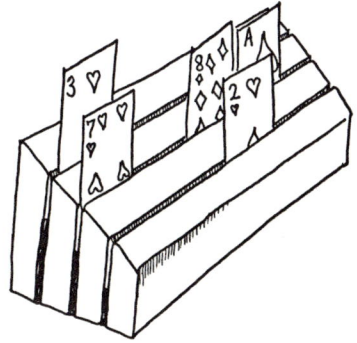

Procedure

Cut the pine into one each of the following sizes and mark in pencil with the appropriate letter:

    a. 9" × 3½"
    b. 9" × 3"
    c. 9" × 2½"
    d. 9" × 2"

Cut the cardboard (to be used as separators) in the following sizes and mark:
a. 9" × 2¼"
b. 9" × 1½"
c. 9" × 1"

The cardboard separators need to be only thick enough to allow a playing card to rest firmly on the surface, but should be securely glued to prevent the card from slipping between the cardboard and wood.

Sand all the pine pieces. With the plane, bevel the top of each 9" length at an angle, planing with the grain. Round off the sharp edges of the top pieces with sandpaper to avoid damage to the cards as they are inserted. Stain or varnish all surfaces.

Glue the strip of cardboard marked "a" between the pine pieces "a" and "b," making sure the cardboard separators are flush with the sides and bottoms of the pine pieces. Glue separator "b" between pine pieces "b" and "c," and cardboard separator "c" between pine pieces "c" and "d." The sides and bottom of the holder should be smooth.

A piece of felt can be glued to the base of the holder to keep it from sliding on a smooth surface and to protect the surface from scratches.

Carving or Chopping Boards

Materials

1. electric jigsaw with heavy blade
2. ¾" hardwood, such as maple
3. vegetable oil
4. latex paint, flat or semi-gloss
5. cardboard or heavy stock paper for pattern
6. drill with ¼"-½" bit

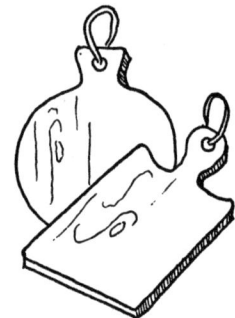

Procedure

Prepare the pattern as shown in Figure 13-88 or 13-89. Mark the outline on the wood, using the straight edge of a piece of wood as guide. Saw the piece, going slowly on curves to prevent blade breakage. Sand the flat surfaces and edge well.

If the non-cutting surface is to have a contrasting color, carefully paint the edges and flat surface on one side with flat paint. When dry, repaint these surfaces with semi-gloss paint.

Drill a ¼" × ½" hole in the top for hanging.

Rub vegetable oil on the cutting surface. Let dry; put a second coat on, rubbing in well.

Craft Projects 243

Figure 13-88 Round Board

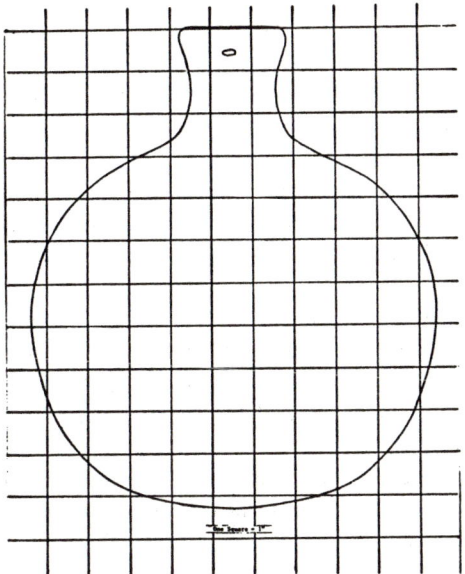

Figure 13-89 Rectangular Board

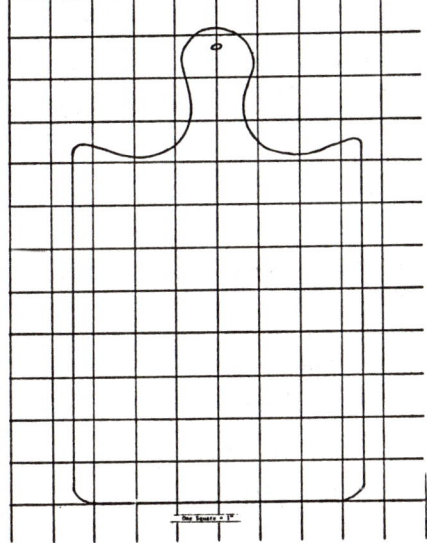

Variations

The non-cutting surface can be decorated in various ways. A small line design can be painted on after the flat paint is applied, such as a family tree, flowers, or animals, then clear varnish can be applied to seal it.

A design can also be put over the final paint coat with stencils. This should be sealed with waterproof finish.

Giant Checkerboard

Materials

1. jigsaw
2. handsaw
3. drill bit, ¼"
4. compass
5. yardstick
6. ruler
7. sandpaper
8. paintbrush
9. glue
10. ½" plywood, 28" × 28" (for board)
11. ½" pine stock (for checkers)
12. ¼" dowels, 2" long (32)
13. red and black semi-gloss latex enamel
14. flat white paint or varnish

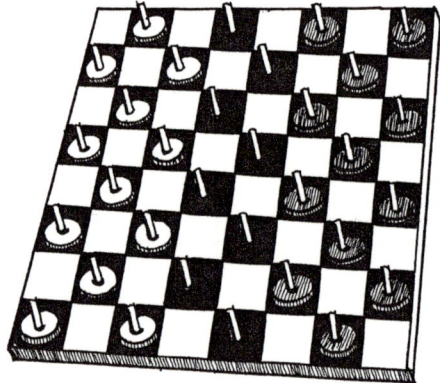

Procedure

Sand the top and edges of the board. Put a primer coat of flat paint or varnish on the entire piece. Mark the board off into sixty-four 3½" squares.

Paint the squares alternately red and black.

When the paint is thoroughly dry, mark the center of each square. Drill a ¼" hole at each center to hold the dowel pegs. Cut and glue the pegs in place.

Cut twenty-four 3" diameter circles from the ½" pine stock. Sand them and give them a primer coat. When it dries, paint twelve checkers red and twelve black. Drill a hole through the center of each checker so it will fit easily but snugly over the ¼" pegs.

Footstool or Child's Bench

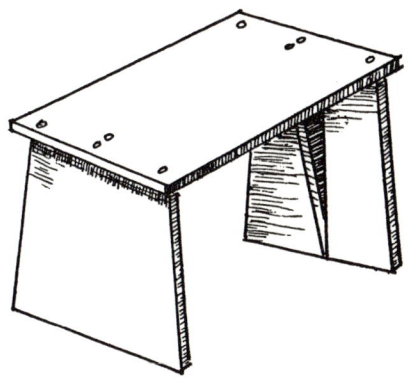

Materials

1. saw
2. hammer
3. screws, flathead
4. countersink bit
5. electric or hand drill
6. screwdriver
7. sandpaper
8. glue
9. wood filler
10. ¾" stock
11. paint or varnish

Procedure

Cut and sand the pieces. Drill and countersink the holes through the first piece of wood so the screws will be flush with the surface of the wood. (See Figure 13-90.)

In assembling, center the side braces on the side supports, or legs, with the top of each brace flush with the top of the side support. The side supports can be aligned flush with the top edges or placed in from the edge about an inch or two.

Cover the countersunk screws with wood filler. Sand when dry. Paint or varnish the completed bench.

Figure 13-90 Foot Stool or Child's Bench

Brace Side

Step Stool*

Materials

1. saw
2. ¾" stock
3. screws, six 1½" flat head
4. screwdriver
5. sandpaper
6. drill
7. countersink bit
8. wood filler
9. paint or varnish

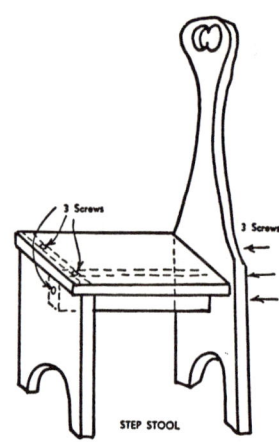

Procedure

Cut and sand the pieces. (See Figure 13-91.)

Predrill the holes as indicated.

Attach the seat and brace to the back, then attach the front leg section. (The seat overlaps a little, forming a ledge.)

Cover the countersunk screws with wood filler. Sand when dry. Paint or varnish the completed step stool.

This stool will help a child reach the sink, or serve as a foot rest for an adult.

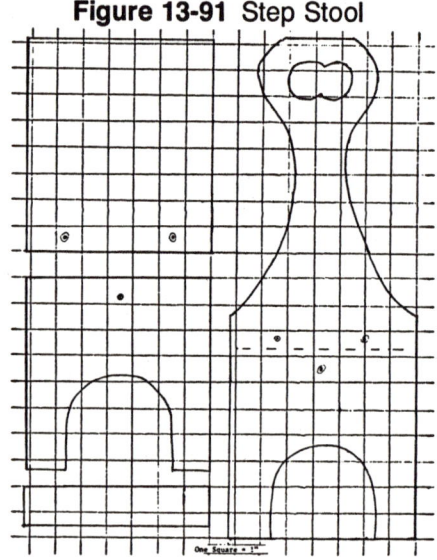

Figure 13-91 Step Stool

*Illustrations are reproduced by permission of S&S Arts and Crafts, Colchester, Connecticut 06415 (Kit W634).

Magazine Rack*

Materials

1. saw
2. ¾'' and ⅝'' stock
3. four dowels, ½'' diameter × 16½''
4. three dowels, ¼'' diameter × 11¾''
5. glue
6. nails, ¾''
7. hammer
8. drill and bits, ½'' and ¼'' (for dowel holes)
9. stain (optional)

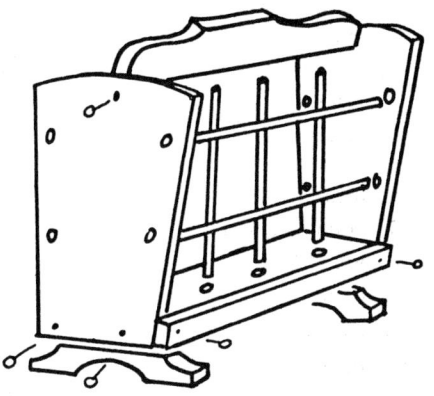

Procedure

Cut and sand the pieces. Drill holes for the dowels as indicated. (See Figure 13-92.) If stain is to be used, stain all the pieces before assembling.

Assembly

1. Glue the four ½'' dowels in the end pieces. (Filing the holes with a round file will help in easing in the dowels.)
2. Center the end pieces on the feet. This will allow a small space on either side for the side strips. Fit the bottom piece between the end pieces. Glue and nail the bottom to the feet and the sides to the bottom.
3. Nail the side strips in place.
4. Glue the three ¼'' dowels in the handle. Glue the dowels into the holes in the bottom.
5. Nail the handle to the sides.
6. Paint the magazine rack if it is not already stained.

---

*Illustrations are reproduced by permission of S&S Arts and Crafts, Colchester, Connecticut 06415 (Kit W639).

Figure 13-92 Magazine Rack

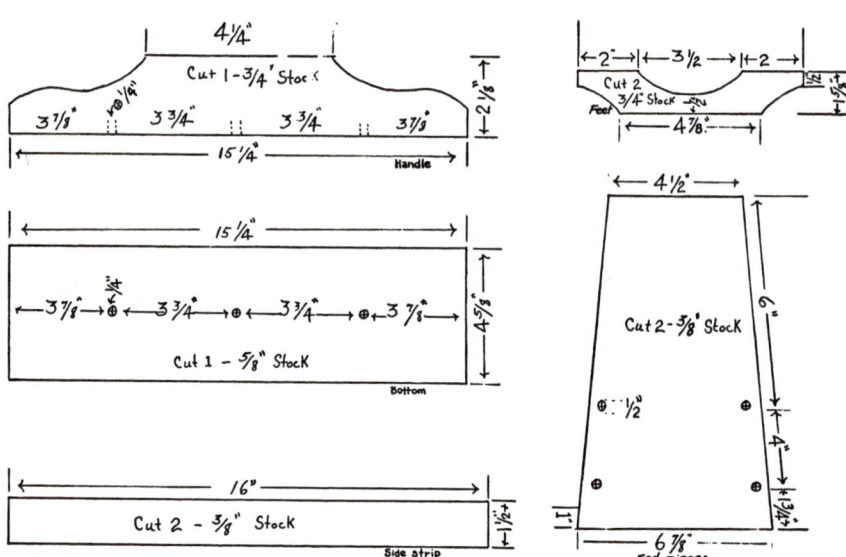

Lap Board

Materials

1. ¼″ plywood or Masonite, 21″ × 24″
2. 24″ strip of hook-and-loop Velcro or leather straps for fastening board to arms of wheelchair
3. shellac or paint

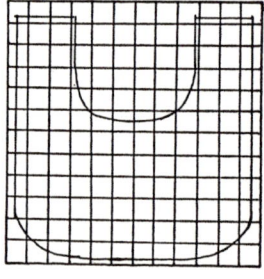

Each Square = 2″

Procedure

Cut the board along the lines shown in the drawing. Sand, then shellac or paint. Be sure the board is smooth to the touch.

Attach the fastenings to the board so the buckle or catching end of the Velcro is on the outside edge of the board. Fastenings can be placed about 1″ down from the top of the arm rest of the lap board.

The depth of the center cutout depends on the size of the user. Measure from the back end of the chair arm; also, measure for the width between the arm rests.

Craft Projects

Inclined Board

Materials

1. plywood for base, pine stock for stops and adjustable arm
2. saw
3. sandpaper
4. screws
5. screwdriver
6. nails
7. three hinges
8. hammer
9. polyurethane varnish
10. paintbrushes

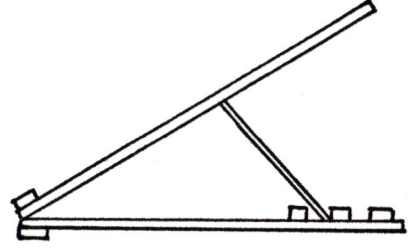

Procedure

After the pieces have been cut (by staff members), sand them well on the tops, bottoms, and sides. Mark the locations for the stops, hinges, and adjustable arm. (See Figure 13-93.) The board can be clear-varnished now or assembled (nail the stops in place, attach the adjustable arm and the top and bottom of the board with the hinges) and then stained or varnished.

Figure 13-93 Inclined Board

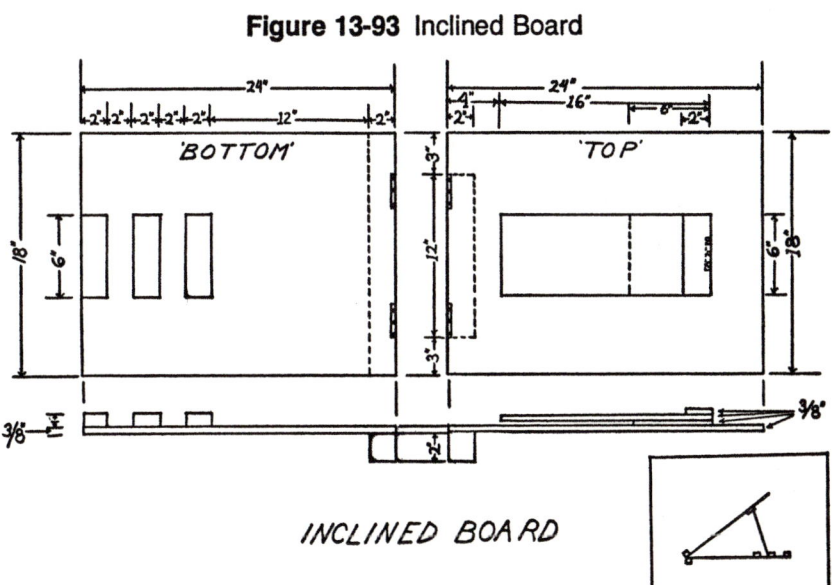

This board can be used with the weighted box for upper extremity exercises. The adjustable angle allows for building up shoulder strength and range of motion by pushing the weighted box up the inclined board. The angle of inclination of the board can be adjusted as the user's strength increases. (Medical recommendation must be obtained before using the board as an exercise modality.)

To keep the board from sliding, self-stick rubber treads can be added to the bottom or the board can be clamped to a table. The board can be used to support or display craft work.

Weighted Box

Materials

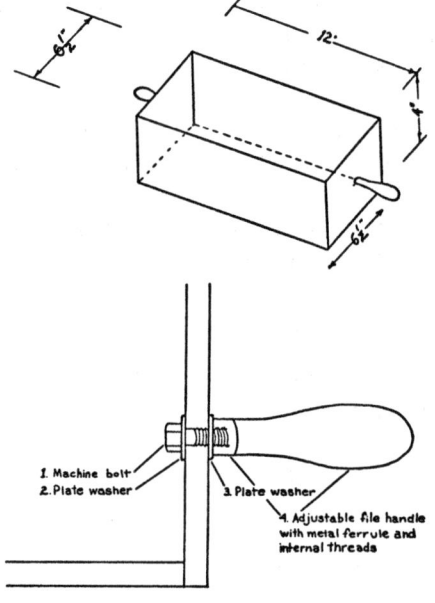

1. ¾" plywood
2. nails and tacks
3. sandpaper
4. 2 adjustable 5" file handles (with metal ferrules and internal threads)
5. 2 machine bolts, 1½" × ⅜"
6. 4 plate washes (½" each)
7. drill bit, ⅜"
8. wrench
9. thread lock glue
10. polyurethane varnish (optional)
11. leather to cover bottom of box and overlap on sides and ends about 1"
12. handsaw or jigsaw

Procedure

Cut wood as follows:

- 1 piece 12" × 6½" for the bottom
- 2 pieces 12" × 4" for the sides
- 2 pieces 6½" × 4" for the ends

Sand and assemble the box pieces. Varnish and let dry (optional).

Drill holes in the center of each end piece. Insert handles and apply thread lock glue, following the directions given on the package. Use the wrench to tighten the bolts securely into the handle threads. Caution: Thread lock glue should be applied only by a staff member.

Cover the bottom of the box with leather, overlapping about 1" on the sides and ends, and tack the leather securely in place. The box should glide smoothly over the surface of the inclined board (see preceding section) or a table surface.

Adaptations

Weights may be placed inside the box for muscle strengthening exercises. For individuals with less strength, use fewer weights.

Sandpaper can be attached to the bottom of the box and it can be used for resistive sanding.

Use of the box for exercise should be approved by a therapist or physician in charge.

A Bilateral Sander (BK 5083) 9" square by 4" deep, with interchangeable handles, is available from Fred Sammons, Inc., Box 32, Brookfield, Illinois, 60513, at $19.95. (Order through a facility or surgical supply house only.) To use this device as a weighted box, remove the snap-on sandpaper and replace it with soft cloth, such as flannel.

A Special Note

If ½" stock is used instead of ¾" stock, cut the wood to the following dimensions:

- 1 piece 11" × 5½" for the bottom
- 2 pieces 11" × 4" for the sides
- 2 pieces 6½" × 4" for the ends

Be sure handle and hardware sizes accommodate the ½" stock.

Paint Can Holders

Materials

1. heavy stock, ½" or thicker
2. jigsaw or handsaw

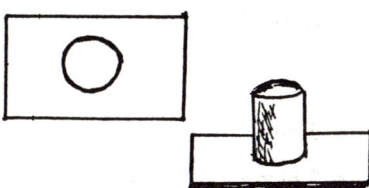

Procedure

Draw a circle on the stock slightly larger than the paint can to be used. Cut along the line leaving just enough space to make it easy to put the paint can in the hole.

Several of these boards can be made to hold the various sizes of paint cans being used.

Use

This holder is a stabilizer for those with poor coordination or with visual problems. For some users, it may be necessary to secure the holder to the work table with a C-clamp.

Workboards for Painting and Drying

Materials

1. heavy stock, ½" or thicker
2. 1½" finishing nails
3. jigsaw or handsaw
4. hammer

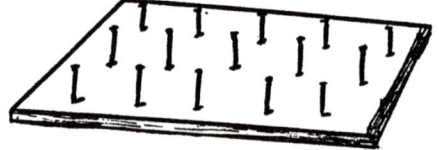

Procedure

Cut the stock to measure 5½" × 14." Hammer the nails into the board, spaced 1" horizontally and vertically.

Use

A board this size will hold small projects to be painted before they are assembled.

If the workboard is placed flat on the table, a piece of work can be placed on top of the nails and painted as the workboard is turned. The work piece can be left to dry, then turned over to finish the underside.

If long periods of drying are needed, several sections of the work can be placed between the nails in an upright or slanted position.

Several such workboards can be made, with the nails at varying distances, depending on the size of the work pieces to be accommodated.

Woodworking Adaptations

- Work can be stabilized with a C-clamp or a vise. (Also see Appendix B for Pony Spring Clamps.)
- In assembling, it is easier to prestart the nails or screws in each piece before assembly. (An awl is used for nails, a gimlet for screws.) If the directions call for staining, it is best to stain the pieces before assembling; stain does not cover the glue used to make the project more secure.
- Kits are available with projects precut and ready to assemble. (See Appendix C for suppliers.)
- Sandpaper can be stapled to blocks of wood of varying sizes for better control while sanding.
- Where glue is called for, it should be allowed to get tacky, before the parts are assembled, to avoid slippage.
- Ratchet screwdrivers can ease the driving of screws for a person with limited strength or range of motion.
- Some tasks lend themselves well to sharing by two or more one-handed participants.
- A crucial factor in the selection of a workbench is making sure that there is adequate clearance for legs and wheelchairs—and no apron on the table. Also, the top surface should be appropriate for pounding. Plastic laminated or wood-grained table tops are not good—solid wood is best.

Bibliography-General

Biegal, Leonard. *The Best Years' Catalogue: A Source Book for Older Americans Solving Problems and Living Fully.* New York: G. P. Putnam's Sons, 1978, $6.95.

Bodkin, Cora; Leibowitz, Helene; and Wiener, Diana. *Crafts for Your Leisure Years.* Boston, Mass.: Houghton Mifflin Co., 1976, $14.95.

Colin, Paul, and Lippman, Deborah. *Craft Sources.* New York: M. Evans and Co., 1975, $12.50.

Cynkin, Sinne. *Occupational Therapy: Toward Health through Activities.* Boston, Mass.: Little, Brown and Co., 1979, $8.95.

Di Valentin, Maria, et al. *Practical Encyclopedia of Crafts.* New York: Sterling Publishing Co., 1970.

Eckstein, Artis Aleene. *How to Make Treasures from Trash: Recycling Can Be Beautiful.* Nashville: The Ingram Book Co., 1972, $8.95.

Family Creative Workshop. *The Golden Family Craft Treasury.* Racine: Golden Press, Western Publishing Co., 1975.

Fish, Harriet U. *Activities Program for Senior Citizens.* Old Tappan, N.J.: Parker Publishing Co., 1971, $11.95.

Gault, Elizabeth, and Sykes, Susan. *Crafts for the Disabled.* New York: Thomas Y. Crowell, 1979.

Glassman, Judith. *New York Guide to Crafts Supplies and National Guide to Crafts Supplies.* New York: Van Nostrand Reinhold, 1975, $14.95 (paper $7.95).

Gould, Elaine, and Gould, Loren. *Crafts for the Elderly.* Springfield, Mass.: Charles C. Thomas, 1976.

Lewis, Sandra C. *The Mature Years: a Geriatric Occupational Therapy Text.* Thorofare, N.J.: Charles B. Slack, Inc., 1979, $9.50.

Mayer, Ralph. *The Artist's Handbook of Materials and Supplies.* New York: Viking Press, 1970.

Moseley, Spencer; Johnson, Pauline; and Koenig, Hazel. *Crafts Designs, an Illustrated Guide.* Belmont, Cal.: Wadsworth Publishing Co., 1962, $14.95.

U.S. Department of the Army. *Craft Techniques in Occupational Therapy* (TM 8-290). Washington, D.C.: U.S. Government Printing Office, 1971, $6.40.

Prices quoted are as of 1979.

Appendix A
Aids for Daily Living

The following list includes only those aids that relate to bathroom and feeding equipment. However, the companies listed handle other self-care equipment, and most of them will send a catalog if it is requested on an institution's letterhead.

Some of the listed items may be referred to by various names, depending on the manufacturer. In some instances, they can also be ordered through a local surgical supply house but may cost more. If the facility does not have a maintenance staff available, it is advisable to order from a company that will install as well as maintain the equipment (particularly bathroom items).

FEEDING AIDS

- **Invisible Food Guard, BK 1115** $5.95
  Large to fit 8½″-10″ plates; clear plastic. To attach to a plate to keep food on it. For those with poor motor control or general weakness.
  Source: Fred Sammons, Inc.

- **Piggy Back Food Guard, BK 1090** $5.45
  Metal, clamps on the back of a plate. The same as the preceding guard but is more adjustable to different sizes of plates and provides less plate coverage.
  Source: Fred Sammons, Inc.

- **Comfort Utensil Holder, BK 1055** $1.60
  For a person with no grasp in either hand. A slot in the holder accommodates a utensil.
  Source: Fred Sammons, Inc.

- **Plastic Handle Swivel Utensil, BK 1014** $4.30
  An adult soup spoon with a built-up handle. For a person who cannot handle food due to poor coordination. The spoon is held level. Similar devices in various sizes and for different utensils are available.
  Source: Fred Sammons, Inc.

- **Dycem Pad, 8" diameter, BK 6570** $4.40
  A stabilizer for putting under plates or glasses. (Available also by the roll or in larger pieces under different order numbers.)
  Source: Fred Sammons, Inc.

- **Scoop Dish, Large, BK 1435** $8.50
  Has a raised edge to give more control, and a lip to push food against. For the weak or uncoordinated.
  Source: Fred Sammons, Inc.

- **Spork, Large, BK 1056** $2.20
  A combination spoon and fork. It is particularly useful with the Comfort Utensil Holder.
  Source: Fred Sammons, Inc.

- **Convalescent Feeding Cup, BK 1254** $2.45
  A covered cup with a hole for a straw. Helps prevent spillage for a person with poor motor control.
  Source: Fred Sammons, Inc.

- **Bilateral Glass Holder, BK 1144** $6.30
  An adjustable glass holder with two handles. For those lacking coordination.
  Source: Fred Sammons, Inc.

- **Cylindrical Foam Padding, BK 6252** $1.60 yd.
  To build up feeding utensils or other items with small handles (paintbrushes, pencils, etc.)
  Source: Fred Sammons, Inc.

BATHROOM EQUIPMENT

- **Suction Brush, BK 6047** $1.35
  A nail brush with suction cups on the bottom. It is particularly helpful for a person who has the use of only one hand.
  Source: Fred Sammons, Inc.

- **Tall-ette I. GJ 1684** $15.00
  An elevated toilet seat (may be known as Hi-John).
  Adds 4" to the seat. Can be easily removed. (May not fit some toilet seats.)
  Source: G.E. Miller, Inc.

- **Toilet Safety Frame, C-4418** $25.30
  Mounts under the toilet seat. Height is adjustable from 25"-29." Assists a person in getting up and down from the seat. Has plastic armrests stabilized on the floor.
  Source: Cleo Living Aids

- **Safety Armrest, C-4420** $65.00
 Is similar to the Toilet Safety Frame, but has armrest sleeves that rest under the toilet seat instead of on the floor. Adds 2" height to the toilet seat.
 Source: Cleo Living Aids

- **Eastern Faucet Handles, H 75314** $7.50 pr.
 These are rigid plastic handles 7" long, which attach to faucet knobs without the use of tools, and make operation easier because of the additional leverage from using the hand or elbow. In sets of two, one red, one blue; each has a Braille symbol to denote cold or hot.
 Source: Maddak, Inc.

Note: Standard bars for wall mounting are available at most surgical supply houses. Installation requires a solid wall or fastening of the bars to wall studs. Because some people need grab support on the right, some on the left, bilateral rails are advisable.

Suppliers for the foregoing items are:

1. Fred Sammons, Inc.
 Box 32
 Brookfield, Illinois 60513
2. Cleo Living Aids
 3957 Mayfield Road
 Cleveland, Ohio 44121
3. Maddak, Inc.
 6 Industrial Road
 Pequannock, New Jersey 07440
4. G.E. Miller, Inc.
 484 South Broadway
 Yonkers, New York 10705

Prices quoted are as of 1979.

Note: The items listed in this section must be ordered through a facility or a surgical supply house.

Appendix B

Activity Equipment

The equipment listed here is suggested for activity programs serving people with physical disabilities.

- **One-Handed Embroidery Frame, 10," C-5009** $12.50
  A holder for knitting, crocheting, and embroidery; most useful for embroidery.
  Source: Cleo Living Aids

- **Rake Knitting Frame, C-5008, 13" diameter** $7.25
  For the one-handed person doing simple knitting. The frames come in a variety of sizes. (This 13" size is suitable for knitting an adult stocking cap.)
  Source: Cleo Living Aids

- **Needle Threader, BK 3505** $.99
  For use by a one-handed person who has difficulty threading a needle but who has good vision. For sewing thread only.
  Source: Fred Sammons, Inc.

- **Left-handed Scissors, BK 6023** $9.50
  For someone who cannot use the right hand for cutting.
  Source: Fred Sammons, Inc.
  Note: Children's blunt scissors can also be used, but only for paper. Electric scissors are useful for a well-coordinated person. Left-handed scissors are also available, in various sizes, in most fabric and notion stores.

- **Scissors for Handicapped, BK 6022** $5.95
  For cutting by those who have diminished hand strength or those whose hand dominance has changed. Has a built-up plastic handle. Also useful for gardening.
  Source: Fred Semmons, Inc.

- **Leather Holding Mitt, BK 5025, Large** $7.65
  To assist people with limited hand strength to hold tools such as sanding blocks, rolling pins, mallets, etc. The mitts come in various sizes.
  Source: Fred Sammons, Inc.

- **Comfort Utensil Holder, BK 1055, Large** (also known as the Universal Cuff) $1.60
  Good for the person having no useful grasp in either hand. It can serve as a holder for small-handled tools, such as paintbrushes, pencils, stamping tools, etc. It is available in various sizes. (This kind of device is easy to make.)
  Source: Fred Sammons, Inc.

- **Suction Brush, BK 6047** $1.35
  To promote independence of the one-handed person in washing. This is basically a nail brush with suction cups.
  Source: Fred Sammons, Inc.

- **One-handed Card Holder, BK 9440** $1.95
  For one-handed people to hold playing cards. This clamps to the edge of the table, plastic discs pinch together to hold cards.
  Source: Fred Sammons, Inc.

- **Type With One Hand Booklet, BK 4031** $1.65
  For the one-handed typist.
  Source: Fred Sammons, Inc.

- **Swivel Bench Vise, 328900000** $15.55
  For attaching to a table for stabilization of equipment and work pieces. (This is available in many hardware stores.)
  Source: Sax Arts and Crafts

- **Sit-on Stitchery Frame, NG 21-05062** $13.99
  An adjustable sit-on frame for needlepoint. Useful for the one-handed or those with generalized weakness.
  Source: Lee Wards

- **Talon Self-Threading Yarn Threader** $.50
  For aid in threading fine or heavy yarn; helpful for those with visual limitations or mild coordination problems.
  Sources: Donahue Sales (and fabric or yarn stores carrying Talon products)

- **Nail-A-Matic, 370-0030** $2.49
  To set nails at an appropriate height, eliminate the need for depth perception, and give a wider surface for hammering. (Use of both hands is necessary.)
  Source: American Handicrafts

- **Adjustable Work Table, GJ 2678** $266.00
  For supporting equipment for work. Can be moved, raised, or set at an angle; has a cutout space for the user.
  Source: G.E. Miller, Inc.

- **Pony Spring Clamps**
  BK 5161 1" opening $1.65
  BK 5162 2" opening $2.65
  BK 5163 3" opening $4.70
  For holding work pieces. Easily used by a one-handed person who needs to secure items to the table.
  Source: Fred Sammons, Inc.

- **Ja-Son Snip Loop Scissors, SL 725** $4.95
  Made with a single plastic spring-loaded loop.
  For those who cannot handle normal scissors because of strength or joint limitations. Designed for light cutting.
  Source: Scott and Fetzer

- **Flower Gatherer H77401** $33.00
  For those who are limited in reach or who can utilize only one hand. A strong, light tool for cutting and gathering flowers. Flat gripping jaws hold the stem of a cut piece until released.
  Source: Maddak, Inc.

- **Weed Puller H77404** $30.00
  For those limited in bending or kneeling. Can be used with one hand. A trigger-operated hand grip closes the jaw when squeezed.
  Source: Maddak, Inc.

Prices quoted are as of 1979.

Suppliers for the foregoing items are:

1. American Handicrafts
   (See local directory for address.)
2. Fred Sammons, Inc.
   Box 32
   Brookfield, Illinois 60513
3. Cleo Living Aids
   3957 Mayfield Road
   Cleveland, Ohio 44121

Note: Most of these items must be ordered through a facility or a surgical supply house.

4. Donahue Sales
   Talon Division of Textron
   41 East 51st Street
   New York, New York 10022
5. Lee Wards
   1200 St. Charles Road
   Elgin, Illinois 60120
6. Maddak, Inc.
   6 Industrial Road
   Pequannock, New Jersey 07440
7. G.E. Miller, Inc.
   484 South Broadway
   Yonkers, New York 10705
8. Sax Arts and Crafts
   207 No. Milwaukee Street
   Milwaukee, Wisconsin 53202
9. Scott and Fetzer Company
   Ja Son Division, Dept. DCI
   217 Long Hill Cross Roads
   Shelton, Connecticut 06484

HOMEMADE AND COMMON ITEMS

- **Spool Holder**

   This device stabilizes thread, lace, or string for an uncoordinated or one-handed participant. The base is cut larger than the size of the objects it is to hold and a dowel in the center holds the spool. The base can be anchored to the table with a C-clamp.

- **Can Holder**

   This tool stabilizes cans while the participant works. It is especially useful for an uncoordinated or confused person. A cut-out circle in the wood base holds the can, and the holder can be clamped to the table. (See directions for making this item in the *Woodworking* section.)

- **Ratchet Type Hand Drill and Short-Handled Screwdrivers**

   These tools are helpful to someone working with only one hand. (An awl or gimlet helps the one-handed person to start nails and screws.)

- **Stabilizers**

   C-clamps, wood vises, clipboards, and beanbags are necessary for uncoordinated or one-handed participants.

- **Lapboard**
  This aid is available commercially and can be easily made. It is useful for those who need arm support when sitting in a chair or for those who have body-trunk instability. The board is also useful where table aprons limit access to the work surface. It can be cut out of ¼'' plywood or Masonite and Velcro tape or leather straps can be attached to the sides for fastening around wheelchair arms to increase stability. (See directions for making this item in the *Woodworking* section.)

- **Needle Threader for Wool and Yarn**
  Directions for making the threader can be found in the *Stitchery* section.

- **Clipboard**
  This is handy for holding writing or drawing paper, and can also be used to stabilize a small needlecraft project taped to a mat frame.

- **Stabilized Nail**
  The nail is hammered through the center of a wooden base, point up. It is useful for shaping clay beads or holding a spool of thread to keep it from rolling, and for anchoring other items, such as the pomander ball (see *Nature Crafts* section).

Appendix C

Craft Supply Companies

The companies listed below offer general craft supplies. Additional information is given where it is useful. Most companies will supply a free catalog if it is requested on an institutional letterhead.

SUPPLIER	PRODUCTS
• Albert Constantine & Son, Inc. 2050 Eastchester Road New York, New York 10461	For advanced wood projects, ask for *Constantine's Wood Catalog/Yearbook*.
• American Art Clay Co., Inc. (AMACO) 4717 West 16 Street Indianapolis, Indiana 46222	Clay, modeling tools, and wheels.
• American Handicrafts*	Kits and leather supplies.
• Art Brown 2 West 46 Street New York, New York 10036	Clay, modeling tools, and wheels.
• Baskins & Sons, Inc. 732 Union Avenue Middlesex, New Jersey 08846	Jewelry findings and supplies. (Clasps, jump rings, earring backs, chains, etc.)
• Beckley-Cardy Company 114 Gaither Drive Mt. Laurel, New Jersey 08054	Art materials.

*Check local directory for nearest location.

- Caron International
  295 Fifth Avenue
  New York, New York 10016

  Yarn, craft kits, and latch-hook kits.

- CCM Arts & Crafts, Inc.
  9520 Baltimore Avenue
  College Park, Maryland 20740

- The Craftool Company
  1 Industrial Road
  Woodridge, New Jersey 07075

  Batik supplies.

- Economy Handicrafts
  50-21 69th Street
  Woodside, New York 11377

  Scratch-art paper, craft kits, and supplies.

- Hazel Pearson Handicrafts
  16017 East Valley Boulevard
  City of Industry, California 91744

  Over 200 "how-to" craft books priced from $1.25 to $2.00, each describing a craft.

- Hunt Manufacturing Company
  1405 Locust Street
  Philadelphia, Pennsylvania 19102

  Speedball silk-screen printing materials (also available at most local art supply stores).

- J & A Handy-Crafts, Inc.
  1078 Grand Avenue
  South Hempstead, New York 11550

  Kits, etc.

- J.L. Hammett Company
  2393 Vaux Hall Road
  Union, New Jersey 07083

  Art and school supplies.

- J.L. Hammett Company
  Hammett Place
  Braintree, Massachusetts 02184

  Clay, glazes, kilns, wheels, cones, and modeling tools.

- Kilns Supply and Service Corp.
  38 Bulkley Avenue
  Port Chester, New York 10573

  Clay, glazes, kilns, kiln furniture, modeling tools, wheels, and cones

- Lee Wards
  1200 St. Charles Road
  Elgin, Illinois 60120

  Supplies and kits (seasonal catalogs available).

- Lily Mills
  Shelby, North Carolina 28150

  Yarn, jute, and cord for weaving, needlework, and macramé.

Appendix C 269

- Macmillan Arts and Crafts, Inc.
  9520 Baltimore Avenue
  College Park, Maryland 20740

  Clay, clay components and chemicals, kilns, ceramic tile, tools, and glazes.

- Magnus Craft Materials
  304-8 Cliff Lane
  Cliffside Park, New Jersey 07010

  Kits.

- Nasco Arts & Crafts
  901 Janesville Avenue
  Fort Atkinson, Wisconsin 53538

  Craft equipment.

- Needles 'N Hoops
  Box 165
  Abington, Pennsylvania 19001

  Large-stamped embroidery kits and "sampler kits" (useful for the visually limited) about $4.00 each.

- S & S Arts and Crafts
  Colchester, Connecticut 06415

  A full line of kits, including woodworking and basketry supplies.

- Sax Arts and Crafts
  207 North Milwaukee Street
  Milwaukee, Wisconsin 53202

  Clay, ceramic tile, kilns, cones, wheels, modeling tools, other craft tools, and equipment.

- Sav-on Crafts
  Box 305
  Miami Shores
  Miami, Florida 33153

  Craft supplies listed in a discount catalog.

- Skil-Crafts Division
  Brown Leather Company
  305 Virginia Avenue, Box 105
  Joplin, Missouri 64801

  Leather, copper, beads, and art supplies.

- Stewart Clay Company
  133 Mulberry Street
  New York, New York 10013

  Clay (including raku clay), kilns, pyrometers, cones, tools, wheels, and glazes.

- Vanguard Crafts
  2915 Avenue J
  Brooklyn, New York 11210

- Walbead, Inc.
  38 West 37 Street
  New York, New York 10018

  Beads, macramé cords, and kits.

Appendix D

Food-Preparation Equipment for the Disabled

Although most disabled people can prepare food with standard kitchen equipment, the limitations of a disability make cooking under ordinary conditions difficult, if not impossible. The equipment in the following list is designed to help disabled people to function more independently. Following the equipment list are sources and a list of cookbooks.

An asterisk (*) indicates those items most frequently used.

EQUIPMENT

- **Suction Cup Boards***
  Paring Board Kit, BK 3098 $2.20
  Includes a plastic corner guard, holding nails, and suction cup feet (but a wood base is not provided). For the use of one-handed, weak, or uncoordinated people when cutting, peeling vegetables or fruit, or buttering bread.
  Deluxe Formica Paring Board, BK 3037 $8.70
  Has a plastic corner guard, suction feet, and nails for stabilizing bread and vegetables.

- **Reachers**
  Better-Grip Wooden Reacher, scissor type, 27'', BK 6105 $8.98
  Be OK Reacher, aluminum frame, trigger action, 27'', BK 6109 $15.00
  Be OK Reacher, same as above, 32'', BK 6107 $16.00
  Rubber-Grip Reacher, aluminum tube, tong type, 30'', BK 6103 $12.95
  These help people with limited reach (up or down) in picking up lightweight items. The first three are light and can be handled easily by a one-handed person or one with weakness or joint limitation. The fourth item has rubber discs on the tips which enable it to pick up and hold objects up to 4''. Normal hand strength is required.

- **Suction-Cup Brush*, BK 6047** $1.35
  Helps a one-handed person in washing vegetables or fruit or in cleaning utensils. This item is useful for both self-care and crafts.

- **Rocking Knife*, BK 1405** $5.20
  Aids a one-handed person in cutting food.

- **Suction Base, PC 7766** $1.00
  Secures bowls or dishes to the table. Good for the one-handed or poorly coordinated; works best on round-bottom bowls and when wet.

- **Apron Hoop, BK 3202** $1.25
  Adapts a waist-type apron for a one-handed person. Eliminates the need for tying the apron.

- **Long Oven Mitts (Barbecue Mitts)** $3.00-6.00
  Available at most hardware and department stores. An essential safety item for disabled people using an oven.

- **One-Handed Can Opener,* BK 3050** $49.95
  Designed specifically for a one-handed person. Adjusts for varying sizes of cans. (Some one-handed people can learn to manage a standard electric can opener.)

- **Wheeled Cart** $15.00 and up
  Available at most department stores. Helps when carrying or lifting is impossible. (Users must be cautioned about danger of relying on a free-moving cart for their own stability.)

- **Foldaway Cart, BK 3246 01 (Gold); BK 3246 03 (Black)** $38.00
  Similar to the preceding cart, but can be reduced in size for narrow doorways.

- **Jar Lid Opener, BK 3086** $3.99
  Assists a person with weakness in the upper extremities, or a one-handed person, in opening jars.

- **Pan Holder,* BK 3010** $7.50
  A good safety item. Stabilizes a pan on the stove with suction cups. Is particularly good for a person working from a wheelchair, or a one-handed or poorly coordinated person. The stabilizer must be positioned before the stove is turned on.

- **High Stool*** About $15.00
  Available at most hardware and department stores. Assists a person with limited standing tolerance in conserving energy. Puts the person at a better height for working at a stove or counter top. (Requires a good trunk balance.) Other choices are bar stools with arms, or a stool with a lower step for foot support.

Appendix D   273

- **Grater with Suction Cup, BK 3294** $3.95
  A good stabilizer for a one-handed or poorly coordinated person

- **Kitchen Shears**   About $3.00
  Available at most hardware and department stores. Assists those who have weakness in the upper extremities or the use of only one hand in opening packages. (Left-handed, as well as right-handed, shears may be needed in a facility.)

- **Pan Strainer, BK 3266** $1.20
  Assists in draining food safely. Latches on top of a pan.

- **Economy Bottle Brush, BK 3229** $2.85
  Useful to a one-handed or weak person in washing bottles or glasses. Has suction cups. (This is the mop type; the more expensive bristle brush is also available.)

- **Over-Stove Mirror, BK 3209** $5.95
  Useful for those cooking from a seated position.

Prices quoted are as of 1979.

EQUIPMENT SOURCES

- BK: Fred Sammons, Inc.
  Box 32
  Brookfield, Illinois 60513

- Kagle: Kagle Surgical Supply, Inc.
  4377 Bronx Boulevard
  New York, New York 10470

- PC: J.A. Preston
  71 Fifth Avenue
  New York, New York 10003

COOKBOOKS

- *Calorie Watchers Cookbook*
  Barbara Gibbons and the Editors of Consumer Guide Publications International, Ltd., 1976.
  Consumer Guide Home Quarterly
  Consumer Guide
  3323 W. Main Street
  Skokie, Illinois 60076

- *Cooking with Betty Crocker Mixes,* Large Type 5th Edition*
  Betty Crocker Kitchens.
     General Mills, Inc.
     Box 6, Dept. 885
     Minneapolis, Minnesota 55440

- *Diabetic Menus, Meals and Recipes* $8.95
  Betty West, Revised 1980.
     Doubleday and Company
     501 Franklin Avenue
     Garden City, New York 11530

- *Easy Ways to Delicious Meals*   Large type Free
  Recipes and ideas for the use of convenience foods.
     Volunteers Service for the Blind
     332 So. 13th Street
     Philadelphia, Pennsylvania 19107

- *Home Management*
  Write to the Library of Congress, Division for the Blind and Physically Handicapped, Washington, D.C. 20542, for a selected list of home management books.

- *Mealtime Manual,* BK 3238 $3.95
  This is written especially for people with disabilities and for the aging. It includes resources for food preparation equipment, techniques for saving energy, adaptations for persons with physical limitations, and recipes.
     Fred Sammons, Inc., 1978.
     Box 32
     Brookfield, Illinois 60513

- *The Art of Cooking for the Diabetic* $5.95
  Katherine Middleton and Mary Abbott Hess
     Contemporary Books, Inc., 1979.
     180 North Michigan Avenue
     Chicago, Illinois 60601

- *The Calculating Cook* $4.95
  Jeanne Jones
  Sample menus for well-balanced meals and explanations of exchange lists are presented.
     101 Productions, 1972.
     834 Mission Street
     San Francisco, California 94103

---

*Single copy free; price for multiple copies on request.
Note: The items listed in this section must be ordered through a facility or surgical supply house.

Appendix E

Aids for the Visually Impaired

Here is a brief list of some aids that have been found useful in activity programs for the visually impaired.

AIDS

- **Magnifying Reader with Stand, BK 3452** $12.89
  For reading or fine craft work. Adjusts up and down. The magnifier can be detached for hand use.
  Source: Fred Sammons, Inc.

- **Extra Large Playing Cards, 4 9/16″ × 7,″ F 71265** $10.00
  For those with limited sight or limited grasping strength.
  Source: Cleo Living Aids

- **Standard Poker Playing Cards, 2½″ × 3½,″ F 71264** $1.75
  Have enlarged numerals for the visually impaired.
  Source: Cleo Living Aids

- **Raised Large Print Telephone Dial, MC 561** $.65
  Has raised, enlarged numerals and letters; fits over a standard dial telephone.
  Source: American Foundation for the Blind

- **Low-Vision Playing Cards, 2½″ × 3½,″ GS 259** $3.35
  Suits are color-coded for players with low vision.
  Source: American Foundation for the Blind

- **Hi-Marks, WS 462** $2.95
  For creating raised surfaces to mark wood, cloth, paper, and metal. Useful for adapting games for easier identification.
  Source: American Foundation for the Blind

- **Checker Set, GS 83** $5.25
  For the visually limited or blind; board is marked with recessed 1" squares; checkers are round for one player, and square for the other.
  Source: American Foundation for the Blind

- **Dominoes, GS 101** $6.95
  For the visually limited. Prominent raised dots identify the blocks.
  Source: American Foundation for the Blind

- **Fiberglass Measuring Tape, SEM 488** $3.25
  Tactile indications are reinforced holes.
  Source: American Foundation for the Blind

- **Right-Line Paper, RLP 101** $16.50
  Narrow and wide rule, 250 sheets each.
  For those who have difficulty in following the lines of regular paper. Made with raised lines superimposed on the printed lines.
  Source: Modern Education Corporation

- **Marks Script Guide, WS295** $17.95
  Allows writing within a ¾" space; a guide moves up and down one line at a time and a margin stop can be moved to the left or right.
  Source: American Foundation for the Blind

Prices quoted are as of 1979.

SUPPLIERS

- American Foundation for the Blind
  Consumer Products Division
  15 West 16th Street
  New York, New York 10011

- Cleo Living Aids
  3957 Mayfield Road
  Cleveland, Ohio 44121

- Modern Education Corporation
  P.O. Box 721
  Tulsa, Oklahoma 74101

- Fred Sammons, Inc.
  Box 32
  Brookfield, Illinois 60513

SERVICES AND RESOURCES

- **American Foundation for the Blind**
  15 West 16th Street
  New York, New York 10011
  Offers the following publications:
  1. *Aids and Appliances*
  2. *How Does a Blind Person Get Around?*
  3. *How to Integrate Aging Persons who are Visually Handicapped into Community Senior Programs*
  4. *Recreation and the Blind Adult*
  5. *Directory of Agencies Serving the Visually Handicapped in the United States*
  6. *Products for People with Vision Problems*

- **Bell Telephone Company**
  (Contact the local business office.)
  Provides telephone aids for the blind at minimal cost.

- **R & R Bowker Publishing Company**
  1180 Sixth Avenue
  New York, New York 10036
  Publishes *Large Type Books in Print*. This index is also available in public libraries.

- **Choice Magazine Listing**
  Dept. MC, P.O. Box 10
  Port Washington, New York 11050
  Provides free subscriptions to selections of 70 publications, on discs, for Talking Books record players.

- **Division for the Blind and Physically Handicapped**
  Library of Congress
  Washington, D.C. 20542
  Provides applications for the Talking Books Program and refers applicant to the nearest cooperating library or agency.

The Division for the Blind and Physically Handicapped in the Library of Congress has developed a collection of braille and recorded materials for eligible readers.

Books and magazines in the Library of Congress program are available on loan, free of charge, to readers via a network of cooperating libraries. Readers may receive cassette machines and phonographs free on permanent loan.

To inform readers of the most recent books and magazines available in the program, the division publishes two bimonthly magazines, *Talking Book Topics* and *Braille Book Review*. Lists of recorded and braille materials are also compiled in several catalogs, including *Talking Books Adult, Press Braille Adult, For Younger Readers: Braille and Talking Books,* and *Cassette Books*. Talking books recorded in Spanish are listed in *Libros Parlantes*.

Eligibility for the program is determined by the inability to see well enough to read a convention print book or the inability to hold a book or turn a page. Individuals who desire service will need a brief statement describing the characteristics of their disability from a competent authority such as a medical doctor, registered nurse, optometrist, professional staff member of a hospital or other institution or agency, or, in the absence of any of these, a professional librarian.

For specific eligibility requirements readers should consult their cooperating libraries, or write to the Division for the Blind and Physically Handicapped, Library of Congress, Washington, D.C. 20542.

from *Talking Books Adult,* 1976-1977

- **Recording for the Blind, Inc.**
215 East 58th Street
New York, New York 10022
Publishes *The News of the Week Review,* as well as tapes, textbooks for college students, and foreign language recordings.

Appendix F
Magazines

Magazines do accumulate! Here is a quick and easy reference system: Write the craft title and page number of articles of interest on 1" × 3" self-adhesive labels and stick them to the cover of each magazine as you scan it on its arrival.

Available by subscription at under $10.00 per year are two nationally popular craft magazines:

- Crafts 'n Things
  Clapper Publishing Co., Inc.
  14 Main Street
  Park Ridge, Illinois 60068
- Decorating & Craft Ideas
  P.O. Box C-30
  Birmingham, Alabama 35283

These magazines have a variety of craft ideas with simple directions, drawings, and illustrations. *Decorating & Craft Ideas* is the more sophisticated of the two; *Crafts'n Things* includes in each issue the best selections from *Pack O'Fun*, a children's craft magazine.

Available nationwide (at supermarkets only) are *Woman's Day* and *Family Circle*. These are monthly magazines, with special-interest issues published at intervals during the year. For information on availability and prices, write:

- Family Circle, Inc.
  488 Madison Avenue
  New York, New York 10022
- Woman's Day
  CBS Publications
  Department PH
  1515 Broadway
  New York, New York 10036

Appendix G

Medical Glossary

ambulatory Walking or able to walk.
aphasia, dysphasia Total or partial inability to use or understand words.
bilateral Affecting or using both sides (both hands, wrists arms, etc.).
cognitive skills The level, quality, and/or degree of comprehension, communication, concentration, problem solving, time management, conceptualization, integration of learning, judgment, and time-place-person orientation.
coordination The ability to perform motions in a smooth concerted way.
deformity Distortion or malformation.
dexterity Skill and ease in performing physical activities.
extension The act of straightening a flexed limb or being straightened.
flexion The act of bending a limb or being bent.
hemianopsia Blindness in one half of the field of vision in one or both eyes.
hemiparesis Slight or incomplete paralysis of one half of the body. (*Hemiplegia* is complete paralysis of half of the body).
kinesthesia The sensation of the position, weight, or movement of the body.
mobility Ease of movement.
perception The ability to interpret sensory messages from the internal and external environment.
prehension The act of grasping.
pronation The turning of the palm downward.
prone Lying with the face downward.
proprioception Awareness of posture, movement, and danger in equilibrium; knowledge of position, weight, and resistance of objects in relation to the body.
residual The remaining function following trauma or disease.
resistive Opposing or counteracting force.
sensation An impression of stimuli, including hearing, smell, taste, temperature, touch, vision, and pain.

sequential Characterized by a sequence; a following of one thing after another; succession.
spasticity Involuntary muscle contraction characterized by increased tension resulting from lack of inhibition. (Spasticity is characteristically found in the anti-gravity muscles, such as the flexor of the arms and the extensor of the legs.)
stereognosis Ability to recognize the form of solid objects by touch.
supination The turning of the arm or hand so the palm is upward.
tactile Pertaining to touch or to the ability to recognize objects or forms by touch.

Bibliography—Crafts

ART

Friend, David. *The Creative Way to Paint.* New York: Watson-Guptill Publications, 1966.

BATIK AND TIE DYEING

Deyrup, Astritch. *Getting Started in Batik.* Riverside, N.J.: Macmillan Publishing Co., 1971, $2.95 (paper).

BRAID WEAVING AND TURKISH KNOTTING

U.S. Department of the Army. *Craft Techniques in Occupational Therapy* (TM 8-290). Washington: U.S. Government Printing Office, 1971, $6.40.

LEATHER LACING

Tandy Leather Company. *ABC's of Leatherwork.* (See the telephone directory for local Tandy Crafts locations or write to Tandy Leather Co., Box 791, Fort Worth, Texas 76101, for location nearest you), $4.00.

U.S. Department of the Army. *Craft Techniques in Occupational Therapy* (TM 8-290). Washington: U.S. Government Printing Office, 1971, $6.40.

NATURE MATERIALS

Appel, Ellen. *Sand Art.* New York: Crown Publishers, 1976, $1.98 (paper).

Epple, Anne Orth. *Nature Crafts.* Radnor, Pa.: Chilton Book Co., 1974.

Miles, Bebe. *Designing with Natural Materials.* New York: Van Nostrand Reinhold, 1975, $10.95.

Peterson, Roger Tory, and McKenny, Margaret. *A Field Guide to Wildflowers of Northeastern and Northcentral North America.* Boston: Houghton Mifflin, 1968.

Squires, Mabel. *The Art of Drying Plants and Flowers.* New York: Barrow Co., 1974.

PAPER AND GLUE

Kenny, Carla, and Kenny, John B. *The Art of Papier Mâché*. Radnor, Pa.: Chilton Book Co., 1968, $4.95 (paper).

Lorrimar, Betty. *Creative Papier Mâché*. New York: Watson-Guptill Publications, 1971.

PRINTING AND STATIONERY

Auvil, Kenneth W. *Serigraphy: Silk Screen Techniques for the Artist*. Englewood Cliffs, N.J.: Prentice-Hall, 1965, $8.50.

Rainey, Sarita, and Wasserman, Burton. *Basic Silk Screen Printmaking*. Worcester, Mass.: Davis Publications, 1971.

Steffan, Bernard. *Silk Screen*. New York: Grosset and Dunlap, 1963, $1.95.

STITCHERY

Bargello

Meyer, Ann. *Bargello Basics*. Leisure Arts Leaflet No. 104 (obtain through local craft or needlework shops), $1.50.

Silverstein, Mira. *Bargello Plus*. New York: Charles Scribner's Sons, 1973, $9.95.

Williams, Elsa S. *Bargello–Florentine Canvas Work*. New York: Van Nostrand Reinhold, 1967.

Embroidery

Coats & Clark Company. *100 Embroidery Stitches*, pamphlet No. 150-A (available in most local variety stores), $ .50.

Dreesman, Cecile. *Embroidery, A Complete Handbook for the Beginning Embroiderer*. New York: Macmillan Publishing Co., 1969, $4.95.

Enthoven, Jacqueline. *The Stitches of Creative Embroidery*. New York: Reinhold Publishing Co., 1965, $7.95.

Guild, Vera P. *Creative Use of Stitches*. Worcester, Mass.: Davis Publications, 1969.

Nichols, Marion. *Encyclopedia of Embroidery Stitches, Including Crewel*. New York: Dover Publications, 1974, $4.95.

Needlepoint

Beinecke, Mary Ann. *Basic Needlery Stitches on Mesh Fabrics*. New York: Dover Publications, 1973, $2.50.

Better Homes and Gardens. *Better Homes and Gardens Needlepoint*. Des Moines: Meredith Corp., 1978, $3.95.

Coats and Clark Company. *Needlepoint Stitches*, pamphlet No. 225-A (available in most local variety stores), $ .50.

Feiner, Wilhelmina Fox. *Adventures in Needlepoint*. New York: Doubleday & Co., 1973, $9.95.

STRING ART

Cunningham Art Products. *Designing in String–String Art Designs for Wall Decor.* The Royal-Craft Library, 1972. (Obtain through local craft dealers.)
Hazel Pearson Handicrafts. *Dimensional String Art, No. HA 20.* (See Appendix C for address.) $1.50.

WOODWORKING

Jackson, Albert, and Day, David. *Tools and How to Use Them.* New York: Alfred A. Knopf, 1978, $8.95.
Sibley, Hi. *Wood Projects.* South Holland, Ill.: The Goodheart Wilcox Co., 1970, $4.00.

Note: Prices quoted are as of 1979.

Index

A

Able Disabled Club, 68
Activities. *See* Craft activities; Craft projects
Aids for daily living, 257-59
American Foundation for the Blind, 76
　braille games and, 78
　marked measuring cups and, 206
　services of, 277
Architectural barriers, 69
Arm function loss, activities for, *13-14, 15*
Art
　activities for, 180-82
　paper and glue, 79-95
　string, 113-16
　therapy value of, 179
Attention span (short). *See* Concentration span (short)
Avocado plant, starting of, 231

B

Bargello (stitchery)
　instructions for, 141, 143-48
　therapy value of, 142
Basins (sinks), useful hints concerning, 51
Bathrooms, 50-51
　equipment for, 258-59
Batik work
　instructions for, 164-66
　therapy value of, 163-64
Beads (creative clay), 203
Bean mosaic kitchen canister, 185-86
Behavioral problems, activities for, *11*
Bilateral Sander (equipment), 251
Blindness. *See also* Braille; Visually impaired participant
　services and resources and, 277-78
　therapeutic activities and, *18,*77-78
Body image distortion, activities for, *21*
Books
　for the blind, 277, 278
　cooking, for the disabled, 273-74
　home management, 274
　Spanish talking, 278
Borrowing of material (supplies), 54
Bottle dipping (container), 169, 171-72
Box (weighted), 250-251
Bracelets (creative clay), 203
Braid weaving projects, 105-108
Braille, 76, 278. *See also* Blindness
Braille Book Review, 278
Brain-damaged participants, food preparation and, 64
Bread dough animals, 197-99

Note: Page numbers in italics designate exhibits.

287

Bread dough wreath, 200-202
Bread making, 65
Bulletin boards, usefulness of, 51
Burlap flowers, 207-210

C

Card holder for playing cards, 241-42
Cardiac problems, windowsill gardening and, 229
Carrot plant, growing of, 231
Carving board, 242-44
Cautions. *See* Safety
Central nervous system dysfunction, hand sawing and, 185
Ceramics. *See also* Clay modeling
   glazing and, 196-97
   therapy value of, 189
   visually impaired and, 77
Chairs (functional), 49-50
Checkerboard, 244
Child's bench (footstool), 245
Chopping board, 242-44
Citrus fruits as house plants, 231
Clay modeling
   glazing and, 196-97
   instructions for, 191-95
   jewelry/dolls, 202-204
   therapy value of, 189-91
Clubs for disabled, 68
Collage, 181
   tissue paper, 79, 94-95
   visually impaired and, 179
Color coding
   activities programs and, 57
   of craft material, 114
   of craft room, 56
   of woodworking room, 55, 238
Communication problems
   activities for, *10-11*
   motivation and, 31
Community aid, 69
Concentration span (short)
   activities for, *9-10*
   horticultural projects and, 229
   modeling with clay and, 191

Confused participant
   activities for, *10*, 111, 164
   art work and, 179
Container decorating, 169-78
Cookbooks for the disabled, 273-74
Cooking. *See* Food preparation
Coordination. *See* Muscle coordination
Cornhusk flowers, 210-11
Cornstarch modeling (creative clay)
   instructions for, 202-206
   therapy value of, 189-91
Craft activities. *See also* Craft projects; Craft room; Group activities; *names of specific craft activities and items*
   demonstrations and, 40
   equipment/supplies for, 53-58, 261-65, 267-69
   goals of, 4-5
   for men, 106, 155, 234
   news publication and, 59-61
   participant evaluation and, 5, *22, 23*
   program operation for, 33-37
   psychological/physical analysis of, 4-5
   record keeping and, 57-58
   safety/material use and, 55
   sample of craft item (importance of), 73
   types of, 5
   uses of, 3-4
   for visually impaired, *18, 20*, 75-78
   volunteers and, 39-45
Craft magazines, 279
Craft projects. *See also* Craft activities; Craft room; *names of specific craft item or project*
   art, 179-82
   batiking/tie dyeing, 163-68
   braid weaving, 105-108
   container decorating, 169-78
   flower making, 207-214
   horticulture, 229-32
   leather lacing, 155-62
   modeling (clay-dough-cornstarch), 189-206
   mosaics, 183-88
   nature materials, 215-28
   paper and glue, 79-95

printing, 97-101
stationery, 97, 102-103
stitchery, 127-54
string art, 113-16
Turkish knotting, 105-106, 109-111
woodworking, 233-53
yarn winding, 121-25
Craft room, organization of, 56-57
Craft supply companies
    (addresses/products of), 267-69
Creative clay. *See* Cornstarch modeling
Crewel work, 129
    enlarging-reducing design and, 137-40
    instructions for, 130-35, 137
    therapy value of, 127-28
    transferring designs and, 141
Crocheting, 127

D

Daily living aids, 257-59
Deafness, activities and, *19, 20*
Decorative containers. *See* Container decorating
Decoupage
    instructions for, 81-82, *83*
    therapeutic value of, 79-80
Depression, activities for, *6-7,* 190, 235
Designs
    enlarging-reducing, 137-40
    transferring, 141
Diet planning, 65
Discarded materials (supplies), 53-54
Disorientation, activities for, *10,* 197
Disruptive behavior, activities for, *11*
Dolls (creative clay), 202-204
Doors, wheelchair clearance and, 49
Dough modeling
    instructions for, 197-202
    therapy value of, 189-91
Dried arrangements, 215, 216-17
Dry skin, clay as irritant to, 191
Drying grasses, flowers, cones, and seedpods, 232

E

Egg carton gardens, 230
Elbow motion, therapy for, 97, 105, 113, 121, 128, 155, 169, 170, 179, 189, 207, 215, 216
Embroidery, 129
    enlarging-reducing designs and, 137-40
    instructions for, 135-37
    therapy value of, 127-28
    transferring designs and, 141
Endurance
    art work and, 179
    horticultural projects and, 229
    limited, activities for, *16,* 97, 121, 163, 169
Equilateral triangle (string art), 117-20
Equipment. *See also* Tools; Supplies
    activity, 261-65
    bathroom, 258-59
    craft room organization and, 56-57
    daily living aids, 257-59
    electrical, caution and, 57
    food preparation for disabled, 271-74
    horticultural, 229
    kitchen, 66
    woodworking room organization and, 55-56, 236-38
Eye patients. *See* Visually impaired participant

F

Fabric flowers, 212-14
Facility
    craft room organization and, 56-57
    furniture for, 49-50
    important factors regarding, 47-48
    kitchen in, 66
    physical features of, 48-51
    woodworking room organization and, 55-56, 236-38
Family
    activity motivation and, 31-32

home activities and, 68
Feeding aids, 257-58
Floors, non-slip and color of, 48-49
Flower drying, 232
Flower gatherer, 263
Flower making, 207-214
Food preparation, 63-66
    cookbooks for disabled and, 273-74
    equipment for disabled and, 271-74
    measuring for, creative clay and, 206
Footstool (child's bench), 245
Frustration (of participant)
    art work and, 179
    modeling with clay and, 190
    working off of, 79, 155
Furniture (facility), 49-50
    workbench, 253

G

Games, 35, 43
    braille, 78
Gardening projects, 229-32
    hanging herb garden and, 239-40
Glazing, 196-97
Glossary (medical), 281-82
Grasses, drying of, 232
Greeting card holder, 121-25
Group activities. *See also* Craft activities; Craft projects; Home activities
    aims of, 25
    batiking as, 163
    bread dough animals as, 199
    bread dough wreath as, 202
    clay modeling and, 189
    decorative containers as, 169
    food preparation and, 63-66
    initiating, 26
    leadership support and, 25, 27, 29
    male (woodworking), 234-35
    nature material work and, 215, 226
    news publication as, 60
    operation of, 26-27
    paper and glue projects and, 79
    printing projects and, 98

project suggestions for, 27-28
tie dyeing as, 168

H

Handedness. *See* One-handedness
Hand function loss
    activities (general) for, *13-14, 15*
    art work and, 182
    batiking and, 163
    decorative containers and, 169-70
    flower making and, 207
    leather lacing and, 156
    modeling with clay and, 189, 190
    mosaics and, 183
    nature materials and, 215-16
    paper-glue projects and, 79-80
    scissor use and, 79
    stitchery and, 127, 128, 149
    weaving-Turkish knotting and, 105-106
Handicraft activities. *See* Craft activities
Handy Handicapped Stroke Club, 68
Hangboard, 238-39
Hanging herb garden, 239-40
Hanging planter, 240-41
Hart, J.A., 75
Head, lack of control of, activities for, *17*
Hearing, importance of to visually impaired, 76
Hearing loss, activities for, *19, 20*
Herb harden, hanging, 239-40
Home activities
    carry-over to, 67-69
    stitchery as, 128
Homemade activity items, 264-65
Home management books, 274
Horticultural projects, 229-32, 239-40
House plants, 229
    hanging herb garden, 239-40
    from the kitchen, 230-31
Hyperactivity, activities for, *12*

I

Inappropriate behavior, activities for, *11*
Inclined board, 249-50

Index 291

J

Jewelry (creative clay), 202-204
Joint diseased
    activities for, 14-16, 127, 128, 163
    horticultural projects and, 229
    modeling with clay and, 189, 191

K

Kitchen (facility)
    features of, 66
    horticultural projects and, 230-31
    stove caution and, 64
Kits (expensive), 54
Knitting, 127
    frame for, 261
    visually impaired and, 77
Knot tying (one-handed), 154

L

Lap board, 248
Large type print. *See* Print (large type, for visually impaired)
Leaf prints, 101
Leather holding mit, 262
Leather lacing
    instructions for, 156-62
    therapy value of, 155-56
    visually impaired and, 77
Leg loss, activities for, *13*
Library Service for the Blind and Physically Handicapped, 78, 278
Low self-esteem, activities for, *7-8,* 191
Lunch preparation (group activity), 65

M

Magazine page art
    instructions for, 91-94
    therapeutic value of, 80
Magazine rack, 247-48
Magazines
    for the blind, 277
    craft, 279
Marbleized paper
    instructions for, 102-103
    therapy value of, 97-98
Mash method (papier mâché), 85-90
Masking tape container, 170, 174
Medical glossary, 281-82
Memory
    and activities to avoid, 105
    braille and, 78
    enhancing, mosaic work and, 184
    poor, activities for, *9-10,* 121
Men, activities for, 106, 155, 234
Mentally impaired, string art and, 113
Mexican jewelry and dolls, 202-204
Mobility problems. *See* Motion impairment
Modeling (clay-dough-cornstarch), 189-206
Mosaics
    instructions for, 185-88
    therapy value of, 183-85
Motion impairment
    activities for, *17*
    paper-glue projects for, 79
Motivation
    clay modeling and, 189
    examples of, 29-30
    methods, 30
    problems of, 30-32
    volunteers and, 40-41
    woodworking and, 233
Muscle coordination, 186
    bread dough modeling and, 202
    decorative containers and, 170
    food preparation and, 64
    kitchen grater for problems with, 273
    lack of, activities for, *16*
    modeling with clay and, 190, 196, 197
    nature note paper making and, 220
    paint can holder and, 252
    paper-glue projects and, 79, 80
    string art and, 113, 116
    woodworking and, 233
    yarn winding and, 121
Muscle strength loss
    activities for, *14-16*
    scissors for, 263
    weighted box and, 251

N

Nature craft note paper, 215, 218-20
Nature materials
  instructions for using, 216-28
  therapy value of, 215-16
Nature plaques, 215, 220-22
Needlepoint
  instructions for, 141, 148-51
  therapy value of, 142
Needle threader (one-handed), 152-54, 261
News publication, 59-61

O

One-handed card holder, 261
One-handed embroidery frame, 101, 261
One-handedness
  art work and, 182
  decorative containers and, 169-70
  hemming (ironed) and, 166
  kitchen grater for, 273
  knitting and, 127
  knot tying and, 154
  lid-opener for, 272
  marbleized paper and, 103
  modeling with clay and dough and, 196, 199, 204
  nature craft work and, 220, 222, 227, 228
  needle threader for, 152-54
  papier mâché and, 88, 90, 94, 95
  printing projects and, 98, 101
  stitchery and, 142
  string art and, 113, 114
  tie dyeing and, 164, 168
  Turkish knotting and, 105
  typing booklet for, 261
  woodworking and, 234, 253

P

Paint can holders, 251-52
Paper and glue craft projects, 79-95
Paper weight, 170, 175
Papier mâché
  instructions for, 83-90
  therapeutic value of, 80
Participants. *See also specific disease category*
  activities profile for, *22*
  activity analysis and, 4-5
  evaluation of, 5, *22*, 23
  food preparation by, 63-66
  home activities and, 67-69
  motivating, 29-32
  perceptual disabilities and, *20-21*
  physical disabilities and, *12-17*
  program operation and, 33-37
  scissor use and, 79
  sensory disabilities and, *18-19*
  social-psychological difficulties and, *6-12*
  volunteers and, 44-45
Patchwork container, 170, 173-74
Paul Klee project (art), 180
Perceptual disabilities
  activities for, *20-21*
  art work and, 181
  batiking and, 163
  bread dough animals and, 199
  color choices and, 187
  mosaics and, 183, 184
  paper-glue projects and, 80
  stitchery projects and, 128
  string art and, 113
Physical disabilities, activities for, *12-17*
Pineapple plants, starting of, 231
Pine cone angel, 215, 222
Pine cone wreath, 216, 223-24
Planter (hanging), 240-41
Playing card holder, 241-42
Pomander ball, 216, 224-25
Potato plant, growing of, 231
Practice circle (string art), 115-16
Print (large type, for visually impaired), 78
  books in, 277
Printing projects, 97-101

R

Recording for the Blind, Inc., 278
Record keeping

craft activity, 57
participant evaluation, 5, *22*, 23
Respiratory problems
   horticultural projects and, 229
   woodworking and, 235

S

Sand terrarium, 216, 225-27
Safety
   activity material use and, 55
   bathroom-kitchen items and, 257-59
   equipment/supplies and, 57
   hot wax and, 163
   supervision (batiking) and, 166
   tool use and, 185, 196, 215, 235
Scissors
   for handicapped, 214, 261
   help with use of, 79
   left-handed, 111, 261
   for strength-loss participant, 263
Scratch art, 181
Seedpods, drying of, 232
Seizures, electric tool use and, 235
Self-esteem (low). *See* Low self-esteem
Self-image (damaged), activities for, *9*
Sensation loss, activities for, *19*
Sensory disabilities, activities for, *18-19*
Setting. *See* Facility
Sevel, David, 75
Shell container, 171, 172-73
Shoulder (impaired), improvement activities for, *15,* 97, 105, 113, 121, 155, 164, 179, 189, 215, 216
Silk screening, limitations of, 97
Skin diseases, clay as irritant and, 191
Smoking, danger of, 55
Social-psychological difficulties, activities for, *6-12*
Spanish talking books, 278
Speech loss
   activities for, *19,* 114, 184
   activity motivation and, 31
   art work and, 179
   card games and, 35

   modeling with clay and, 190
Staff
   education for, 36-37
   electric tool supervision and, 235
   jigsaw supervision and, 215
   modeling with clay and, 190-91
   motivation and, 30-32
   news publication and, 60-61
   occupational therapist, 33
   operation of groups and, 26-27
   part-time, 32
   sense of failure and, 30-31
   supervision of hand sawing and, 185
   volunteers and, 39, 41-42, 45
Stationery projects, 97, 102-103
Step stool, 244
Stone painting, 216, 227-28
Stool
   foot (child's bench), 245
   step, 244
Storage units, 50, 55
Stove, caution concerning, 64, 66
Strip-dip method (papier mâché), 83-85, *86*
Styrofoam printing, 97, 98
Supplies. *See also* Equipment
   borrowing of, 54
   craft room organization and, 56-57
   discarded materials as, 53-54
   news publication, 59
   woodworking room organization and, 55-56, 236-38

T

Tables, 49
   adjustable work, 263
   kitchen, 66
Talking Book Topics, 278
Telephone
   aids for the blind, 277
   public, necessity of, 51
Television, 51
Terrarium (sand), 216, 225-27
Therapeutic Activities Participant Profile, 22

Tie dyeing
  instructions for, 167-68
  therapy value of, 164
Tile hot plate, 186-87
Tissue-paper collage
  instructions for, 94-95
  therapy value of, 80
Toilet safety items, 258-59
Tools. *See also* Equipment
  craft room, organization of, 56-57
  electric, caution and, 57, 215, 235
  safety and hand saws, 185
  use of, by poorly coordinated, 196
  woodworking, organization of, 55-56, 236-38
Training
  of staff, 36-37
  of volunteers, 42
Transportation, 68
Trunk
  lack of control of, activities for, *17*
  motion, therapy for, 97
Turkish knotting, 105-106, 109-111
Twine wrapping (container), 169, 173

U

Utensil holder, 262

V

Vegetable blocks, 97, 99-100
Ventilation, 50, 186, 191
Vision field loss, activities for, 18
Visually impaired participant
  activities for, comments on, *18, 20*
  aids for, 275-78
  collage work and, 179
  color choices and, 187
  crocheting-knitting and, 127
  decorative containers and, 170
  flower making and, 207
  fragrance garden for, 229
  leather stitching and, 156
  measuring cups and, 206
  modeling with clay and dough and, 196,
  199, 202, 204, 206
  mosaics and, 184
  paint can holder and, 252
  paper-glue projects and, 80, 94
  pine cone wreath construction and, 216
  pomander ball making and, 225
  print type and, 59
  printing projects and, 98
  projects for, 75-78
  stitchery and, 128, 142
  string art and, 114
  tie dyeing as poor activity for, 164
  weaving-knotting and, 105, 111
  woodworking and, 234
Volunteers
  potential problems with, 43-45
  recruitment of, 40-41
  role of, 39
  selection of, 41-42
  training of, 42
  transportation and, 68

W

Weaving
  braid, 105-108
  visually impaired and, 77
Weed puller, 263
Weighted box, 250-51
Wheelchair users
  architectural barriers and, 69
  basin (sink) use and, 51
  bathrooms and, 50
  doors and, 49
  horticulture and, 229
  kitchen and, 66
  kitchen pan stabilizer for, 272
  tables and, 49
  telephone (public) and, 51
Windows (facility), 49
Windowsill garden, 229
Wishing well container, 170-71, 176-78
Wood relief, 187-88
Woodworking projects
  adaptations for, 253

instructions for, 238-52
precautions and, 185, 196, 215, 235
setting up shop for, 55-56, 235-38
therapy value of, 233-35
Woodworking room
  organization of, 55-56
  setting up shop for, 235-38
Workbench, 253
  adjustable, 263
Workboards for painting and drying, 252
Wrist (impaired), improvement activities for, *15*, 155, 169, 189, 207

Y

Yarn winding, 121-25

MAYVIEW STATE HOSPITAL
BRIDGEVILLE, PA. 15017